Immunity Strong

Boost Your Natural Healing Power and Live to 100

Robert G. Lahita, M.D., Ph.D.

Humanix Books

IMMUNITY STRONG
Copyright © 2022 by Robert G. Lahita
All rights reserved

Humanix Books, P.O. Box 20989, West Palm Beach, FL 33416, USA
www.humanixbooks.com | info@humanixbooks.com

Humanix Books is a division of Humanix Publishing, LLC. Its trademark, consisting of the words "Humanix Books," is registered in the Patent and Trademark Office and in other countries.

Disclaimer: The information presented in this book is not specific medical advice for any individual and should not substitute medical advice from a health professional. If you have (or think you may have) a medical problem, speak to your doctor or a health professional immediately about your risk and possible treatments. Do not engage in any care or treatment without consulting a medical professional.

ISBN: 9-781-63006-195-1 (Hardcover)
ISBN: 9-781-63006-196-8 (E-book)

Printed in the United States of America
10 9 8 7 6 5 4 3 2 1

Contents

*Dedicated to my loving wife
and artist, Carolyn D. Palmer*

A Note from Dr. Bob . . . and Dr. Lahita

Greetings, I'm Dr. Bob! Thank you for joining me on this journey through immunity and your immune system, or what I call your biological soul. In the pages of this book, my goal is to give you a different way through stories and metaphor into understanding your immune system—how it works and connects to everything you do, its strengths and weaknesses, and its physical and, yes, spiritual sides. As Dr. Bob, I tried to keep things as simple as possible, but I did not shy away from the science or "dumb it down." That's because I am also Dr. Robert G. Lahita. Dr. Lahita uses the same medical terms people in the profession use and likes to cite lots of important and interesting studies and scientists. As a doctor and scientist, it is important for me to approach the material both ways and be precise. So, I did not hold back on the depth of each chapter's dive. But Dr. Bob knows Dr. Lahita can get really "inside baseball" when it comes to all this immunology stuff. So, for ease of reading, this book is not filled with the footnotes and parenthetical citations that make scientific literature so hard to read, let alone understand. Nor will you find dozens of pages of bibliography for the hundreds of sources

I consulted. In order to keep things readable and also update you with any new findings after the book is published, I have placed all of that and more on my website: *doctorboblahita.com*. The only footnotes in the book will be stories and additional information Dr. Bob or Dr. Lahita thinks you might find fun, informative, or interesting as you read. Finally, Dr. Bob and Dr. Lahita both know they could never include everything about the immune system in one book—at least not one anyone would want to read, let alone carry. This is my take on the biological soul, based on my decades as a doctor, and both sides of me hope you enjoy the journey.

Life, not death, has no limits.

—Gabriel Garcia Marquez

Introduction: Your Biological Soul

A few months before COVID-19 began its relentless push across the globe, I was talking with my wife, Carolyn, over breakfast about the body's immune system. Carolyn was used to these conversations. She knew what she was getting into when she married a doctor and professor of medicine and a microbiologist who had studied civilizations' responses to viruses. That day, I was contemplating how every immune system is unique due to immutable internal factors like genetics and biological sex, as well as external factors like the environment, stress, and the life that is around, upon, and within us: parasites, bacteria, and viruses. But while every immune system works differently to battle everything from the common cold to life-threatening viruses, I also noted a similarity I saw in every patient facing an illness—something like a life force working to keep them alive.

That's when I noticed Carolyn, a sensitive artist, looking at me in a way that usually means "it's time to shut up now, Dr. Bob." Instead, she looked at me thoughtfully and said, "You mean a biological soul?"

Yes! Our immune systems are incredibly complex biological forces that determine our wellbeing. They want to protect us and make our lives long and healthy. They are always at work without our knowing or thinking about them, and they affect how we eat, sleep, work, breathe, and look. As a physician, I have always felt a need to integrate the spiritual, scientific, and emotional factors that enlighten immune function. That morning, after decades of studying the wonder and mystery of immunity, I finally had a name for this great protector that is chiefly responsible for our longevity: *the biological soul.*

According to philosophers, the human soul is dualistic: there is a physical soul and a spiritual soul that integrate to form the foundation of a long life. The same is true of our biological soul, the root of our immune system. The physical (the tangible and measurable) side of this immune system integrates our organs and manifests itself through the biology of the body. It is in our circulatory functions and beating hearts, the manifestations of sex and libido, the functions of the brain, and most importantly, our immunity.

Most people understand the need to take some form of action, like proper diet or exercise, to ensure that this physical side of the biological soul endures and to try to obtain overall happiness. But feelings of happiness are not controlled solely by our physical body, so why should we think that about our immune systems? Because in the past, discussions of a mind-body connection have been relegated to the fringes by medical practitioners, if not dismissed entirely. Today, data, not just supposition, supports this vital mind-body relationship when it comes to immunity. Emotional events that affect behavior, like the death of a family member, the stress of divorce, or an intractable disease are all known to influence immunity negatively and can result in disease and/or a decreased life span through lowered resistance to infection and susceptibility to disease. Meanwhile, positive spiritual actions, such as yoga, meditation, walks in nature, and faith and prayer can increase immunity by ensuring happiness, allowing our bodies to flourish and work to lengthen the life span.

Of course, it is much easier to understand how the physical side of the immune system is critical to life. How staph or strep infections that corrupt the immune system are beaten back with the assistance of modern medicine. How aggressors that destroy the immune system like human immunodeficiency virus (HIV), which cripple immunity, allow opportunistic infections to wrest life from the soul and kill the patient. How organ failure, infertility and arrested reproduction, and possibly behavioral diseases are related to immune dysfunction. From dementia to heart disease to cancer, every day I see patients with disease in which immunity is involved directly or indirectly. Each of these diseases leaves a scientific footprint to motivate me and other physicians toward new directions for research and new ways to treat illness.

But there is much that we still cannot explain. So much of our biological soul operates beyond the physical, without our knowledge. For example, *autoimmunity* (the process in which the immune system attacks the body) has no known cause but could be the result of a novel and yet unknown infection, disruption of *biomes* (organisms that tell the immune system if something is friend or foe), or an anomalous mind-body connection. The study of immunology has grown exponentially to consider all these possibilities, and the development of new therapeutics from this mind-body understanding has made life better for all of us. If there is a Grand Design, this is it: the union of the scientific and the spiritual—the mind-body connection in the beauty of our biological soul, its commonness between us, and the vital role that it plays in our lives.

Helping you understand all of this—to nurture the physical and the spiritual and to keep them strong to optimize our lives and boost our body's healing power and help our biological soul live to 100 as it wants to do—is the reason I wrote this book.

Too many of us have limited knowledge of the human immune system—how it works, does not work, and why. The biological soul is complex stuff, and I want you to be aware of and embrace all this complexity—the sacred substance of life—to enhance and prolong your life and give you a greater respect for the similarities rather than the differences between us. More than a metaphor, the design of our populations, the body politic, protective networks, and humanity's common needs mirror the marvelous design of the human body. Together they form a universal spiritual connection to all that we do and who we are.

We are in the midst of a medical and scientific revolution in which our life spans can be increased only with a thorough understanding of, and respect and care for, our biological soul. Our collective destinies are determined by the realization that this soul is affected by forces beyond our comprehension, which in turn are affected by how we care for ourselves and each other. While the biological soul of every person may be different, we are all created with the same components, like snowflakes are to snow.

By cultivating our soul's protective mechanisms, we can guarantee ourselves and our children healthier and longer lives. That is what I mean by "immunity strong": integrating the hard science and data about the immune system with its spiritual side is the master key to unlocking medical miracles of the future—for ourselves and our children. And it starts with you. Whether or not you can optimize your life and boost your body's healing power moves from the inside out and derives its strength from listening to yourself.

To paraphrase a great philosopher, reading is thinking with someone else's brain instead of one's own. I invite you to think with me and change your life.

1
The Response Team Inside You

Corliss, a young woman pregnant with her first child, had *systemic lupus erythematosus*, which had produced skin lesions and pain from her inflamed heart and lungs. Lupus can be lethal during pregnancy, and in Corliss, it had caused her immune system to attack her body, a process that we call *autoimmunity*. Autoimmunity mostly occurs when the immune system is tricked by a virus, but no known virus causes lupus. Still, Corliss was nothing but positive and determined to fight for her life.

— * —

Patricia suffered from rheumatoid arthritis. She had stiffness and such severe pain that she was "in pure hell" for about seven hours after waking up. She felt she was always in slow motion. These are standard symptoms of rheumatoid arthritis, which is caused by the immune system mistakenly attacking the body, and in Patricia's case, her joints. A young mother of three, the only time Patricia had felt fine was the three times she had been pregnant. Otherwise, despite the love and support of her husband and daughters, the swelling and pain was constant. "I want to be pregnant all the time," she said. "That's when the arthritis disappears."

— * —

Greg came to the ER complaining of fever, nausea, pain all over, diarrhea, and a rapid pulse. He tested positive for COVID-19. But because the amount of oxygen in his blood was normal (97 percent), he was sent home to self-quarantine for 14 days. Six days later, Greg was back in the ER, gasping for breath and coughing. The amount of oxygen in his blood had dropped to 70 percent and he had to be attached to a ventilator and intubated. A chest X-ray revealed a "whiteout" in both lungs (a lack of air which shows up on the X-ray as the obliteration of air space) caused by a *cytokine storm* in which his immune system was suddenly attacking his organs, one of the most prominent causes of death in the pandemic that resulted from this virus. With concern about blood clots forming, Greg was given blood thinners and injected with steroids to shut down his immune system. There was no way to know if he would regain consciousness, let alone survive.

— * —

Corliss, Patricia, and Greg—just three of the thousands of patients I have seen in my practice, in clinical studies, and on hospital rounds for nearly half a century. All of them suffering, sometimes very acutely, from unrelenting pain. All of them depending on the strength of their immune systems—what I call their biological soul—to survive. From the time I first began my medical career, people like Corliss, Patricia, and Greg have compelled my compassion and my curiosity. What is the ailment? What causes it? Why is it happening to that particular person? Why are they suffering from it more or less than others? What can I do to alleviate it? The answer to these questions lies in the root of the biological soul. While everyone's biological soul is specific to that person and his or her family, understanding how it works in co-ordination with all of the other organs of the body is our first step to answering these questions and all the questions in this book.

This chapter lays out the basics of and explores the magnificence of the immune system and its inner workings, which I liken to your body's protection network or first responders. This is the foundational information you need for understanding what immunity strong means throughout this book and appreciating just how extraordinarily complex your immune system is. Some physicians, scientists, and other colleagues have chafed at my attempts to simplify the presentation of this complexity with only occasional digressions when necessary. This is exactly why the immune system remains a seemingly impenetrable mystery. My goal is to make the purpose of this incredible system approachable without minimizing the complexity, shying away from more technical terms, or acknowledging just how much is left to understand by those who study it.

THE IMMUNE SYSTEM: YOUR FIRST RESPONDERS

Imagine your body as a huge city. When your city is humming along, everything is in sync and balanced. Your organs are communicating well with each other. You are in a condition called *homeostasis*. Homeostasis is what your body wants. If homeostasis is maintained, life continues. But just like a real city, life isn't so simple. Things can go wrong, sometimes very wrong, and when they do, your immune system is your city's first responders—your law enforcement, paramedics, EMTs, firefighters, SWAT team, and more—policing your body and ready to answer the call when there is a problem or danger, large or small.

The biological origins of your first responders are your *embryonic stem cells*—cells that give rise to all others in the body like the white blood cells that protect your city against crimes attempted or perpetrated by infections and foreign invaders. Your liver metabolizes the nutrients needed to provide these first responders with just the right amount of energy and vitamins to ensure good health. Your *biomes*, which naturally inform the immune system what is friend or foe and work together to strengthen it, are providing the first responders all the support they need to be efficient when unwanted parasites, bacteria, and viruses appear.

Some embryonic stem cells begin their training as first responders before birth in your bone marrow (B cells), and others in glands like the thymus (T cells) or organs like the lung or liver (*monocytes*). Eventually all of them will "graduate" and know when to provide the city of your body with two types of protections: *innate response* and *adaptive response*.

Innate response is the closest thing your body has to an "automatic" response to *antigens* or viruses, bacteria, or parasites or that enter your body from the outside. Antigens are criminals—petty thieves, mass murderers, and everything in between that lurk around and in the underworld of your body's city. Some are violent and attack quickly. Others take their time and move slowly. Many of these criminals are stupid and are easily caught by your innate response and eliminated without you ever knowing. Your innate first responders see and/or feel something isn't right and launch a forceful attack. This attack neither depends on the expansion of other cell types nor has any memory or recognition if or what kind of culprit is involved. It only knows how to differentiate between something that belongs in your city (self) and something external affecting it (nonself).

Sometimes you do see and/or feel your innate response. For example, when you get a splinter in your finger, your innate response is pain, inflammation, and redness. When you catch the flu, your innate response is fever and an upset stomach. When a virus touches your skin or is inhaled, your innate response sounds the alarms internally to protect your organs and, hopefully, catch the bad guys before they can do much harm. Calling these signals "alarms" is appropriate because the medical name for the signal that causes this response is *alarmin*. Alarmins and defensins (proteins known as *pattern recognition receptors*, which are common to other species like flies and cockroaches and are prehistoric sensors for immune systems in all living creatures) call together a cellular and chemical response involving as many as 200 different signals and receptors. They are the hotline to all your first responders, moving quickly to alert the rest of the body. This ancient human system of pattern recognition relies on the barriers of skin, gut, and mucous membranes of the respiratory tract and a sophisticated system of communication between cells of all varieties (much more sophisticated than those of actual first responders within a true metropolis).

When the antigens are too difficult for your innate first responders to handle, they sound the alarm for more help. That's when your adaptive response team arrives on the scene. Adaptive response works days after the innate response to determine whether or not a foreign substance was previously known to the system. Adaptive response is led by millions of T and B white blood cells we call *lymphocytes*. Lymphocytes are made in the bone marrow from stem cells that are always cruising around in your blood. They are carefully located in certain organs and called into action by *antigen-presenting cells* (APCs) that trigger your immune response to attack the criminal cells. APCs are monocytes—*macrophages, dendritic cells,* and some B cells—that serve as your immune system's central command. The B cells are your rank-and-file police and tactical team "on the ground," maturing into plasma cells to produce Y-shaped proteins called *antibodies* that "handcuff" the bad guys and mark an antigen for destruction. They then process offenders and inform T cells and others to take further action.

The process of your immune system's recognition and arrest of an antigen (or a fragment of it) begins with the receptors found on T and B cells (each coded by different genes). T cells control most of what goes on in both innate and adaptive immune responses in part by activating the cells that destroy criminal invaders. They are the special forces and detective division of the immune system wrapped into one—communication experts, investigators, and directors of how crime scenes within the body are handled. They mature in the thymus gland (hence the "t")—the city hall of the immune system—and coordinate with other cells to launch direct attacks on the criminals.[1]

The immune system is like a rheostat (the type of light switch that can brighten or dim your lights in the dining room) for T cells—controllers of activity that can alert natural killers or helpers. Things like drugs, hormones, vaccines, and metabolic processes turn the rheostat up or down, as do certain diseases where the immune activity and your immune system needs to respond with antibodies or enhanced cellular immunity. The rheostat is controlled by your metabolic processes and by *cytokines*.

Cytokines are one family of a pair of powerful chemicals that form the communication network of your immune system called the *biological regulatory system*: cytokines tell cells what to do and *chemokines* tell cells where to go (like a 911 call). Cytokines and chemokines are sent by the T cells with a message to destroy criminals like a highly trained SWAT team. T cells make a substance called interferon which helps provoke natural killer T cells and serves as a first-line defense against viral infections. These natural killer T cells can destroy other cells infected with specific markers on their surface. T helper cells are divided into two groups: type I helper (TH1) T cells and type II helper (TH2) T cells. Both have critical roles to play in attacking antigen criminals. TH1 T cells are the special forces division. They help macrophages or the antigen-presenting B cells make antibodies in response to the criminal invasion through specific cytokines. TH2 T cells help B cells make antibodies through additional cytokines. These T cells survey the crime scene and ask, *Who is or isn't welcome in the body?*

All in all, T cells do their job brilliantly, including producing those cytokines that regulate everything. When your adaptive response is successful, you begin to feel better. And here's even better

---

[1] B cells get their "b" name from glands in chicken bowels called the "Bursa of Fabricius." There is no comparable gland in the human bowel, though there is lymphoid tissue in the human bowel called *Peyers patches* that could be the evolutionary version of the Bursa.

news: Unlike your innate response, your adaptive response does have a memory. It stores an invader's identification in its genetic database for use later to produce antibodies if there's another attempt to attack your body. Your adaptive response is not just part of the first responder team—it's your immune system's criminal database!

Consider a patient of mine who presented with a simple *diverticulum* or bulge in the bowel. Something—probably a fragment of stool or an undigested piece of food but maybe something else that shouldn't be there—had lodged itself in the large intestine, leaving organisms within the bulge with no place to go (called *outpouching*). The result was a collection of pus or large numbers of bacteria and lots of responding white cells forming a small round mass called an *abscess*. The patient's innate response was pain and swelling as bacteria entered the wall of the intestine and then the bloodstream. Then came the adaptive response. Since this patient had had multiple episodes of minor inflammation over many years, the adaptive response was familiar with these bowel bacteria and mounted an all-out fight against the organisms encapsulated in the abscess. After four days, all hell broke loose: APCs commanded the T cells to act, which in turn informed the B cells.

Soon, copious amounts of antibody were being made, all to ward off the infection and protect the body. *Neutrophils*, the most common *phagocytes* (white blood cells which also include monocytes and macrophages that assist in the T cell fight), swarmed the scene as back up for the T cell SWAT team and engulfed the germs. Neutrophils carry special enzymes and set up the bacterial capture and the required chemical assistance for the immune system. In other words, they eat germs and carry them away like the paddy wagons of the immune system. Meanwhile, the patient's cytokines communicated with the lymph nodes (which are like police precincts around your body) around and within the bowel where there are pockets of lymphocytes. The chemokines then allowed the cells to enter the area and they facilitated the inflammatory process while keeping all channels of communication open. The abscess grew as the adaptive response grew. There was fever, pain, and probable bowel obstruction due to swelling and a bowel that was in shock. All first responder resources were now coming to the aid of the patient.

Amazing and dramatic action, right? It's as intense on the inside of your body as it would be on any hospital drama about first responders outside the body. And this is happening every day inside most of us! That doesn't mean the immune system prevails—or doesn't need help. If this was fifty years ago, the end to this patient's abscess episode might have been a sad one. Back then, depending on the patient's age and overall health, the patient could die from the aggressive immune response that resulted from something called *sepsis* (infection of the blood). Today, a surgical opening of the abscess and use of antibiotics assist the immune system in overwhelming the infection to avoid sepsis—as long as the patient sought the help its first responders needed from the human first responders who serve us so well every day. The only problem is when the criminal is not immediately identifiable or even something new.

WHEN A NEW CRIMINAL INVADES YOUR "CITY"

Most of the time when your first responders need more help than they can provide, they alert your brain to call for help through a doctor, hospital, or pharmacist and get the medicine they need to keep working. When a virus or disease is identified in enough "cities," scientists can figure out how to help your first responders deal with them through treatment or vaccines, which often stop the crime before it even has a chance to start, or at least minimizes its impact. But when there is no one to call for help or no one knows how, there is always the possibility that your immune system may not be strong enough to ward off the infection, leading to severe illness, an attack on multiple organs, and death.

This is especially true when a virus is new.

Viruses our immune systems have never seen before can cause chaos, especially when the criminal isn't seen as such. Some viruses trick your immune system into doing something it shouldn't. For example, treating patients during the 1980s for HIV, we saw rare Kaposi's sarcoma cancers resulting from the sudden loss of T cells and the entry of a virus that would normally be defeated (likely a herpes virus). We eventually learned the HIV virus had tricked the men's immune systems to replace the T cells that would normally fight off HIV with those infected by the virus.

Other viruses are sneaky and hide themselves from your first responders, entering your cells before your body has a chance to recognize that a crime has been committed—or believing there is even a crime at all. That was the issue with COVID-19—a stealthy nonliving menace that can use your cells to propagate.

Coronavirus is not uncommon. It is one of many causes of the common cold (another you might have heard of is rhinovirus). The bad thing is that we continually get colds, even after infection, which can mean your immunity to this family of viruses can be very fleeting. And when it comes to a wily and aggressive coronavirus like COVID-19, with infected people showing no symptoms, it can be easily transported to other people who are not as lucky. The result can be what the world just suffered through: a global pandemic.

COVID-19 antigens operate like organized crime syndicates and not only fool the immune system from blocking its functions at every turn, but also cause your immune system to turn on *you*. Your body's T cell killers may be dedicated to antiviral activities through evolution, but even they can be fooled—and like human first responders can sometimes mistakenly go after the innocent. When faced with something like COVID-19, since there is no recognition of the criminal, your adaptive response could go all out in its response, destroying one or more organs (usually the kidney or the lungs) while trying to eliminate the criminal—the biological equivalent of throwing everything at it but the kitchen sink. In doing so, your immune system overreacts and can get so excited that it attacks tissues and cells in your kidney, brain, heart, or in the worst case, in your blood vessels. In other words, it believes your body is the criminal.

This is very different from what happens in an organ transplant when the immune system sees a new lung or kidney as a foreign-based threat, and the T cells are still using the genetically driven protection system for your original organ. That results in a degree of acute rejection of an organ in every transplant in the first three weeks after the procedure. Modern medicine knows how to treat that response with immunosuppressive drugs—the same medication used to treat something as common as asthma or as severe as Corliss's lupus and Patricia's rheumatoid arthritis. These medicines allow the immune system time to accept a new antigen in the form of a donor organ that must be as close an genetic match as possible (from a brother or sister as an example). But when your immune system suddenly believes your body is the criminal, the result is *autoimmunity*, which is what happened in Corliss.

Many of us in medicine believe that the way that autoimmunity develops and produces hundreds of diseases is through a stealthy, effective, brilliant viral infection. Luckily, autoimmunity isn't common and can be treated with revolutionary anti-cytokine drugs or *engineered monoclonal antibodies* (the name for some now-familiar drugs used to suppress the immune system, which act like cortisone but are nothing like that steroid hormone). For example, in cases of severe eye disease, a patient is treated by an infusion (yes, an injection in your eye) of monoclonal antibodies or man-made proteins that block a specific cytokine and allow a person to see. But when resourceful criminal masterminds like COVID-19 attack and cause our cytokine communication receptors to go haywire, healthy people like Greg can end up fighting for their lives through a *cytokine storm*.

A cytokine storm is a full-blown misguided attack by your immune system on your organs, and the most common cause of death in patients infected with lethal foreign viruses. It's like your first responders get brainwashed to turn on you—the biological equivalent of an internal insurrection. Criminals take over your city and order is not easily restored, even with immunosuppressive drugs helping your first responders "deprogram" from the brainwashing. In fact, it is often chaos; and in the worst cases, everything in the body—heart, lungs, kidneys, brain—is rejected. This is why we often heard stories like Greg's during the COVID-19 pandemic: people going from leaving the hospital to being on a ventilator and, in many cases, dying.

In Greg's case, his immune system was being tricked to release an increased number of cytokines to destroy lots of normal cells in the lung, heart, kidney, and even his brain. His immune system's first response was robust: Every one of his first responders from paramedics to the SWAT team rushed to deal with the situation. Cytokines transmitted messages as white cells, along with phago-cytes, which responded, as did his killer T cells, all producing mas-sive degrees of inflammation and fever in an effort to alert his body that something was wrong. There was rioting in the lungs as cells abounded, producing a layer of fluid from inflammation that oxy-gen could not cross. Breathing then became difficult because the normal function of the lung cells had been destroyed. His lungs filled with pus and small mini clots formed to prevent the passage of oxygen across the lung's membranes. COVID-19 had fooled Greg's immune system into all of this. If it got to perform its final trick— the multiple mini clots clogging the very small vessels of the lung (the pulmonary arterioles and venules)—Greg would die. Not that the virus wanted Greg to die. It wanted to use Greg to pass itself on to another host. Dying is almost a final act of altruism to end the suf-fering and save other "cities." (Now you know why zombie movies are so scary to immunologists: the host dies but the virus lives on!)

Long before Greg and COVID-19, I had seen this same progres-sion in Parker, an 18-year-old male who suffered from a cytokine storm caused by a different virus. His lungs filled with fluid. His liver and kidneys were failing. He had a high fever and *anemia* (a significant lack of red blood cells). In the same way the im-mune system rejected a new organ, Parker's immune system was essentially rejecting his entire body, turning on itself by produc-ing defensive antibodies to almost every protein in his body. Near death, Parker was treated by shutting down his immune system with immunosuppressive drugs. I call it the "maximal provocation" of the immune system. There's nothing worse, which is why it is a last resort. Because of his age, Parker survived but not without many sleepless nights for me. I worried the same way about Greg and all the COVID-19 patients suffering from cytokine storms.

After two weeks in a comatose state, Greg's life took a turn for the better. His ventilator was removed, and he slowly regained consciousness. While he was unconscious, his immune system, with the assistance of medicine, was at work connecting all of his organs to communicate once again. His biological soul was back on track and getting stronger—strong enough so he could begin his rehabilitation at home. But there was more than medicine involved.

THE ROLE PLAYERS OF YOUR BIOLOGICAL SOUL

For Greg, the survival of the immune system or its ability to rob him of life, despite its good intentions, depended on how his first responders had been "trained" before the crime was ever committed. So does yours, every day—and not just in matters of life and death. Your genetics, immune system's limitations when it comes to infections, environmental factors, biological sex, how your first responders communicate, any vaccines administered, the organisms or life in and on you, and even how your brain developed all play roles in your biological soul.

For example, you probably know that your genes can increase the chances of developing specific diseases, such as diabetes and heart disease. In the city of your body, your genetic markers are the manual your first responders follow for responding to invading criminals. Your killer T cells are often guided by immune heredity. They use a specific receptor protein to identify their role in your immune system and to define the roles of T and B cells in circulation. Among the many things the inherited receptors do is help distinguish "foreign" from "self," and the inheritance of these markers either allows or prevents anything foreign from proliferating within your body. Sometimes it is clear from genetics that these receptors make someone susceptible to infections and viruses like TB, strep, staph, or COVID-19. But I and other medical professionals have been left scratching our heads as to why perfectly healthy people succumb to parasites, bacteria, or viruses that are usually harmless and why blood relatives often succumb to the same innocuous things.

How people respond to infections probably date back generations to an early great grandmother or grandfather. In the case of how people handle infections like measles or COVID-19, I call it a "crap shoot." Once the recognition occurs in the next generation, there is a flurry of communication informing the lymph nodes and millions of other cells within the immune system through cytokines and chemokines that they must work together to destroy the invading criminals. But in some people, there may be something called *inborn errors of immunity* or another genetic problem that is not immediately apparent until a major infection like a novel coronavirus enters the system. For example, in the COVID-19 pandemic, deaths weren't predictable, but it was obvious that in some people, the availability of cytokines, cascades of antibodies, and immunological genetics were causes of patients' deaths. Their immune systems could have been influenced by many factors like age and *comorbidities*—a bad heart, chronic obstructive lung disease, severe asthma, and those diseases related to obesity based on body mass index. During the height of the pandemic, we also considered the blood types of individuals that placed them at risk (type O was the best to have). But a person could also be young and healthy like Greg with no risk factors and have a genetic predisposition to the virus, allowing it to hijack normal cells in the lungs, heart, kidneys, and other organs and use them to hide and reproduce.

Time will tell how we come to understand COVID-19, but one thing is certain: genetics alone didn't determine everyone's immune response or come close to stopping my medical head-scratching when it comes to why the immune system reacts the way it does in some people and not others. There are so many factors. You could be susceptible to an infection like TB or cholera depending on where you live (prominent in the slums of Delhi and refugee camps in southern Syria). Genetic adaptation might also play a role in the process like it does in susceptibility to malaria, one of the world's deadliest infections. It was overcome by a simple genetic error causing sickle cell disease in some people of African heritage: because of this genetic change, their blood took on a sickle shape that prevented the malaria organism from infecting red blood cells.

The innate and adaptive response of your immune system is also impacted by something else: how you live your life. Stress, diet, exercise, external threats, metabolic influences (alcohol, drugs, etc.), and a host of other factors have proven to interfere with the workings of your immune system via something called *epigenetics* or how your behaviors and environment cause changes that affect the way your genes work.

To me, however, there is no more interesting area within immune diseases than the role of gender and sex. It is often said, "you can pick your gender, but not your sex," and I believe that. Gender is how you choose to identify. Sex is biology—male and female—and changing that biology is harder than simply changing your appearance, how you dress, and the pronouns you use. Gender is a personal option, but it has no effect on genetic-directed immunity. The biological sex you are born with remains a major determinant for everything else in your body's city: cell types, response efficiency, antibody character, and sensitivity to those cytokines and chemokines. That goes for your immune system as well, which may explain why many viruses affect men and women differently or sometimes just one or the other; why women often had more adverse reactions to COVID-19 vaccinations than men; and why men with COVID-19 died sooner than women with the virus.

In fact, I'll go one step further when it comes to sex: I believe there are special aspects of the female genetic makeup, which have to do with having a baby, that explain why women live longer than men—namely, that the immune systems of women are honed to perfection for reproductive purposes and their XX chromosomes contribute to that. Carrying a fetus in a woman's womb is tantamount to carrying a tissue transplant; the baby cannot be rejected in a normal pregnancy because the mother's biological soul tells the mother that the baby, even though its genes are 50 percent from the father, must be protected and retained at all costs. In fact, the whole body must be protected, which is why so many diseases go into remission during pregnancy. Diseases like Patricia's rheumatoid arthritis, which disappeared only to burst back on the scene with a vengeance after each of her deliveries.

I could go on with the wonders of pregnancy and I will, but I am getting ahead of myself. Forgive me; I do that sometimes. I find all of the main roads and side roads of this city so wonderful and fascinating, and I hope you will, too. There is so much more to cover when it comes to genetics and biological sex and all we have talked about so far, and we will cover them and many more major players in your biological soul in helping it and us live to 100. For now, I hope I have hit a nerve with the whole concept of a biological soul and the idea that your body is a city full of first responders. I want you to be fascinated with your own body and gain a deeper respect for your life and all its complexities. I want you to realize there is more to you than you think and have a deeper sense of a part of you that each of us share regardless of belief, age, sex, gender, where we live, and how we behave. I hope to help you look differently at or at least more informatively and mindfully about that vaccine you are getting or the medicine you take.

Remember: immunity strong is not just about action—what you do and how you live—but how much you understand.

Before we move on, however, I want you to know that while making you immunity strong and boosting your body's healing power from the inside out is the goal of those chapters and this book as a whole, we all will eventually die. When someone dies, those left here to remember us often talk about our souls going to a better place. We do not mean our biological souls. We often fail to consider the spiritual side of our immune system, which has been as responsible for our day-to-day existence as the physical side. Call it what you will—a biological soul, your body's first responders, or just the immune system—it has the power to add to your life or terminate it in a matter of hours. It shows us time and time again how precious and fragile life is, how each of us can come to an end with a simple bacterium or a novel virus. To understand it, we must acknowledge the relationship between the spirit, the mind, and the body in making that immune system strong. We must respect the awesome beauty of its design and appreciate the sacred aspect of this intricate and marvelous system, which can work in concert to prolong our lives.

I see the importance of this mind-body-spirit relationship every day in my patients. I saw it in Greg before and after his rehab—in his spiritual desire to show us that COVID-19 wasn't going to take him as one of its victims. I saw it in Patricia, whose immune system shut down her rheumatoid arthritis while she carried three beautiful babies to term. I saw it in Corliss's endless reserve of positivity despite the physical challenges of her lupus—positivity I believe that transferred to the fetus in her womb, touching both mother and daughter. She fought on through the pain of her disease and gave birth to a healthy baby girl. That girl became an exceptionally gifted child, reading by age three and writing by age four, and defying the odds, Corliss lived to see her become a teenager. Her positive thinking gave the spiritual side of her biological soul remarkable power—power and limitations that we are working every day to understand and control.

DR. BOB SAYS

To help you digest the material, throughout this book, "Dr. Bob" boxes like these will appear regularly to point out essential information. For now, the most essential thing to do is look in the mirror and consider the following questions when it comes to being immunity strong.

- How have you thought about your immune system in the past? Has that changed as you have gotten older?
- Have you or your family members thought more about your health and death because of COVID-19, cancer, HIV, or other infections?
- Have you ever thought about the spiritual side of this biological soul? Why or why not?
- What steps, if any, have you taken to boost your immune system in the past? Why? Why do or don't you feel those steps worked?
- What aspects of the immune system are you most interested in moving forward and why?

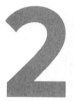

2 Biomes
Life in and on Us

When I was in college, I fell in love with Theodor Rosebury's *Life on Man.* It captivated students like me who were smitten by biology and fascinated by the organisms around us that become part of our bodies. But neither Rosebury's book nor any of my medical training prepared me for one of my more memorable early days as a doctor. A colleague and I were set to perform a routine colonoscopy on a ninety-year-old woman. Our nurse had assured us that this patient had been prepped, meaning that her bowel had been cleared of any stool and we were ready to go. We turned out the lights, advanced the scope, and saw what can only be described as a tsunami of stool coming toward us. *Oh crap!* (Well, explosive diarrhea, to be specific.) My colleague yelled for us to run but it was too late. When we turned the lights on, the two of us looked like dalmatians in our all-white doctor suits.

Telling this story always gets a laugh, along with a bit of a gag reflex or juvenile snigger, from an audience, but I use it to make an important point: I couldn't run from poop then, and we can't in this book either. Poop, especially someone else's, may not be great to get on you but it is a great way to get into those organisms that still fascinate me and have as much to do with your health than anything else in life: *biomes* or communities of microorganisms or microbes within and on you. When it comes to biomes, you are never alone: From before you are born, they are present everywhere in and on your body and work together to strengthen your immune system and tell it if something is friend or foe. Think of them as a kind of immune system moral compass.

Bacteria are the most dominant players among your biomes and make your poop as much a living thing as a mass of dead cells and waste. In your gut alone, there are roughly 100 trillion biomes from your small intestine into your large intestine, meaning that there are also trillions of genomes that belong to bacteria visiting your body, along with millions on our skin, and many more within our lungs, mouth, and urinary, genital, and reproductive tracts. Gut bacteria play a role in regulation of immunity, development of the nervous system, and are your main source of vitamin K and vitamin B complex. It should come as no surprise then that these bacteria and all your biomes are deeply affected by what you eat. Yes, you are what you eat, as well as what you interact with, the environment around you, the stress you feel . . . and your biological soul knows it. In fact, biomes are essentially your biological soul's soulmates, only with names you cannot pronounce and microscopic forms that look like worms and peas.

Biomes are an evolutionary marvel that have allowed us to travel to various parts of the world since the dawn of man; places where there was low oxygen at high altitudes, extreme heat, limited or unusual food sources, and so on. They permitted genetic adaptation, for example, allowing people with dark pigment from warmer climates an ability to regulate their blood pressure and heart rate as they migrated to colder parts of the globe. Most importantly, the biome was the environmental variable that allowed us to thrive and support defenses against infection, pain, and early death. They informed the immune system and allowed it to develop and adapt to the dangers of the environment. It is very likely that the immune system in early *Homo sapiens* was largely regulated by the biome. If there was malaria, cholera, and a whole host of other infections from environmental change, biomes eventually allowed humans to adapt and formed a natural deterrent to death from these infections.

So, it is amazing how little we think about them today—or see them as a danger and try and get rid of them. Simply put, our physical *and* mental wellbeing depends on our biomes thriving within and on us. While this chapter speaks almost exclusively to biomes of the gut, research may eventually show biomes of other areas like the skin might be just as important to the immune system as the bowel. Digesting what this means—not just taking action to change certain aspects of your diet and your behavior—is the subject of this chapter and the next key to becoming immunity strong.

THE DOWN AND DIRTY OF DIRT

Howard Hughes, the mid-twentieth-century American businessman, went from billionaire playboy to world-famous recluse and obsessive-compulsive germaphobe. He believed his neighbors made him sick by living unkempt lives, demanded that anyone who touched his food use layers of paper towels (and that most of that food was contaminated anyway), and yet still believed that everything was covered with a small layer of dirt that no amount of cleaning would help. I think all of us who lived through the global pandemic may have some understanding of Hughes's need to socially distance from others, and stories of bacteria leading to food poisoning should make us all be conscious of safely handling our food. But the dirt part is harder to get my head around.

If I saw one of my children eating dirt, playing in the cat box, or wrestling with the dog, I was sorry for whoever was doing laundry but took comfort in the fact that they might be arranging their adaptive immune system to respond to horrid infections later in life. Robust collections of healthy bacteria in a child's bowel can build immunity at a young age that lasts through a lifetime. In other words, children who eat dirt, pick their noses and eat the snot, and luxuriate in covering themselves in mud, might have healthier immune systems *because* they do that.

As counterintuitive as all that sounds, studies of rural children who wallow and even swallow dirt when they are little reveal that they are less prone to allergies that affect suburban and urban children. Children living on a farm, being around and breathing in (and likely ingesting a bit of) manure have less allergies and healthier immune systems. There is also evidence in adults of being "dirt happy," meaning playing in and laying in dirt acts as a natural antidepressant and mood lifter. This is something we continue to study but think about that the next time you resist the urge to lie on the ground. Howard Hughes be damned—the power of dirt might be the best thing for training immune systems!

DR. BOB SAYS

Don't ignore the power of dirt! Your bowel uses the abundance of bacteria in and on the body to inform the immune system. The biomes of the bowel, as well as your skin, lung, and gastrointestinal tract, have effects on many bodily functions. They are a welcome community of organisms with their own genes and essential to good health—and have been since our ancestors began to migrate around this planet, allowing them to adapt to new environments.

There is growing evidence that this power of dirt starts the moment we are born. This is called the "Hygiene Hypothesis."

According to the U.S. Food & Drug Administration, the Hygiene Hypothesis "suggests that the critical postnatal period of immune response is derailed by the extremely clean household environments often found in the developed world." Exposing babies and young children to certain biomes in dust and dirt protects against allergies and antigens (the criminals from Chapter 1). It strengthens their immune system's tolerance to antigens the same way they strengthened the immune systems of our nomadic ancestors. By contrast, denying the child's exposure weakens their immune system's tolerance. Antigen exposure at a young age essentially enlarges a child's biomes and creates a robust immune system that can result in reduced effects of respiratory diseases like asthma and resistance to allergic diseases like eczema.[1]

All we just covered makes biomes *adjuvants*, or substances that increase your immune response to an antigen. Biomes are also adjuvants that assist anything that stimulates the immune system like vaccines. They do this through the flora of your bowel and your cell's genetic library. As we will cover in Chapter 7, most vaccines contain materials like aluminum to prod the immune response as adjuvants, but these organisms within your bowel are an endogenous or inner stimulant for the immune response. I saw this in the lab when germ-free mice (sterile mice born without exposure to any organisms and fed sterile diets) were immunized with the influenza virus, and they failed to mount an immune response. A similar response was found in the mice that were given huge doses of antibiotics and had their bowels chemically sterilized.

Okay, take a breath, lie down in the dirt, and contemplate all of this before we do another gut check.

---

[1] No one has explained the high rates of asthma and allergy among the urban poor children in America. Studies suggest that traffic related pollutants from auto exhaust and the aerosolization of automobile rubber tires along roads and highways are responsible for a 12 percent increase of asthma in children by age 40. I can only imagine that such pollutants affect every biome of the child's body.

DR. BOB SAYS

The food you eat and the drugs you ingest—such as the indiscriminate use of antibiotics to treat nonexistent bacterial infections like the common cold—can alter your biomes and change your immune responses to many things, including vaccines, which are not as effective in those with altered biomes.

FROM YOUR INSIDE OUT OR YOU ARE WHAT YOU EAT

"You are what you eat" is an expression usually deployed as an insult—a joke made at the expense of others about their diets by those asserting their healthy diets and fitness. But it's no joke. What you eat has major effects on you, something the originator of the phrase, the renowned nineteenth-century French gastronome Jean-Anthelme Brillat-Savarin in *Physiology of Taste*, understood when he wrote: "Tell me what you eat, and I will tell you what you are." It has been two centuries since Brillat-Savarin made connections between the external (social and political) and internal (anatomy, histology). Yet many of us still struggle to make this connection ourselves and *act* in spite of all the scientific advances in understanding the biomes within and on us.

The 27 feet of bowel we all have helps us to digest food and absorb it. It degrades complex fats, carbohydrates, and proteins and gives you energy. But it is also part of the protective network of the body since it prevents the colonization of harmful organisms from gaining a foothold. This microbe-host relationship is vital to our wellbeing and is thus deeply affected by diet. Research has revealed unambiguous and startling differences in the health and effectiveness of gut microorganisms of thinner versus obese people. Studies for decades have shown that your diet can increase or decrease the risk of cardiovascular disease in both men and women, which is the most common cause of death in developing countries. Yet our food chain remains as much about class, politics, and calories than what might be right for you—and be doing to you inside and out.

While food and diet research and debate are constantly evolving, we need another gut check as the health of the communities of organisms essential to our biological souls hangs in the balance—something that antibiotics not only cannot fix but can also hurt. I never understood this more than the day I met Melanie.

Melanie's abdominal pains felt "like she was being punched in the gut every five minutes." Each volley of pain would be followed by a burst of watery diarrhea. She had suffered these indignities for a period of days. In taking her medical history, we learned Melanie had been on antibiotics for a urinary tract infection for some weeks and developed her bowel problem only recently. That's when we realized she was suffering from a serious—and deadly—infection caused by a bad bacterium *Clostridium difficile*, or *C. diff*. *C. diff* causes inflammation and severe damage to the bowel. It is particularly insidious as it can reoccur weeks after treatment and in some cases can be fatal. Melanie was already heading in that direction when we saw her, and her diarrhea was only making her weaker. In her case, this treacherous opportunist bacterium also took advantage of a bowel in which most of the normal flora had been killed by her antibiotics and then kept taking advantage when the new round of potent antibiotics used to treat it kept killing her biomes.

To be sure, any disruption of the bowel wall results in invasion of bad organisms and the subsequent inflammation, but Melanie's case was an extreme version of a not uncommon problem (more than half a million people get *C. diff* every year), and one which is quite serious in a time when antibiotics are prescribed by doctors without regard for a patient's biome. Melanie had few options left, so we deployed the exact reverse of the story that opened this chapter: through a colonoscopic procedure, we transplanted stool in capsule form from a patient who had normal healthy flora *into* Melanie's bowel in order to try and reseed her bowel with those normal biomes.

As a medical student, I can recall my microbiological mentor at Jefferson Medical College, Dr. Russell Schaedler, growing *aerobic* organisms (those that need oxygen to grow) and *anaerobic* organisms (those that grow without oxygen and produce a lot of gas). They had bizarre names, smelled horrible, and were in retrospect some of the earliest studies of the biome. Dr. Schaedler knew these organisms had a role to play in normal physiology and homeostasis. Even then, he felt that immune diseases like rheumatoid arthritis and lupus might be connected to the organisms in one's diet. (Joint pains from the gut? Yes!) Other doctors followed. For example, an early paper from Dr. Jose Scher at New York University found that people with rheumatoid arthritis were more likely to have the *Prevotella copri* organism in their intestines. He felt that changes in the body's ecosystem with the rampant and inappropriate use of antibiotics was one possible cause of the rise of autoimmune diseases in general. Dr. Scher also researched a nagging condition called psoriatic arthritis in patients and found that yet another unusual bug common to normal stool was absent in the bowels of those patients.

All these bugs have strange names—many unfamiliar to most microbiologists, let alone laypeople—and make for impressive tongue twisters for academic discussion. Back then, I only knew one thing: these organisms were exceedingly difficult to grow in the lab, especially the ones called anaerobes that grew in the absence of oxygen. Today, growing these organisms and the cultivation, use, and study of human stool can be big business and a lifesaver for people suffering from *C. diff* and much, much more. For Melanie, unfortunately, it was too late. Her symptoms were too advanced by the time we saw her, but stool transplants do have a cure rate of 90 percent for extreme cases of *C. diff* and further demonstrate the power of poop.

The most important question, however, is not what poop can do to cure disease, but what you can do to keep a balance of healthy biomes inside your bowel before that poop ever comes out. And that brings us back to diet.

It is hard, even impossible, to keep up with the latest fad diet and even the long-established studies of how what we eat affects us. But research consistently shows a diet of meat, rich in sugar, and replete with processed foods can adversely affect the balance of these microbes in the gut and support the extraction of calories from food. A plant-based diet may be more sensible, providing fiber and vitamins without all that sugar. Research has also shown that long-established diets like the Mediterranean or Atkins that steer this way will decrease chances of inflammation as a result of what we eat. Studies in mice suggest that obesity is dependent on the biome of their bowels. A lean mouse given a stool transplant from a fat mouse results in the lean mouse gaining tremendous amounts of weight in a short period of time.

What I advocate for is balance in everything you eat that fits your lifestyle. I do not think vitamins and other nutritional supplements can supply what you don't eat or undo the damage of what you do. But there are practical ways to use diet to eliminate the hyperimmune state and make you immunity strong and boost your immune system, particularly *prebiotics* and *probiotics*.

- *Prebiotics* are microbes that you ingest to encourage the growth of healthy microorganisms like bacteria or yeast that boost the health of your gut and your health overall. They are not digested by your gut but metabolized by the gut bacteria and can change the course of atherosclerosis, type 2 diabetes, and possibly even correct behavioral issues. They can be found naturally in food sources such as onions, garlic, leeks, asparagus, bananas, chicory root, and dandelion greens. Many consider foods with fiber like barley and oats as great prebiotic foods as well.
- *Probiotics* are friendly bacteria that restore your gut flora. Certain foods like yogurt, sauerkraut and kefir, tempeh (a fermented soybean product), kimchi (Korean fermented cabbage), miso (a Japanese seasoning), kombucha (fermented tea), pickles, traditional buttermilk, natto (another fermented soybean product),

and many kinds of cheese are natural probiotics for your gut. All of these can boost immune function by way of biomes.

For most people, the inclusion of probiotics is a natural thing. Use of prebiotics may take a little planning and thought. Consider this and any information you read carefully as you look at what you eat and any modification of your diet. Millions of people around the world believe in the use of probiotics, and while they are not tested in rigorous scientific trials, there is substantive evidence that the ingestion of these probiotics is safe. Just be careful to check claims on packaging to be sure you are getting more of the good stuff and less of the sugar and processed substances used to transport them. There are also prebiotics and probiotics which can be prescribed by physicians and nutritionists.

All in all, what should be clear is achieving longevity of your biological soul must include your diet and the biome of the bowel, which have been teaching your immune system good from bad since and before you were born.

DR. BOB SAYS

Everything you ingest affects your biology for better or worse, but it particularly affects your immune system. For better, prebiotics and probiotics should be included in your diet several times per week. For worse is not just about diets heavy in trans fats and processed foods, but also includes the indiscriminate use of antibiotics that can make you very sick and even kill you if left untreated.

BIRTH AND BIOMES

Your bowels are sterile before birth; microbial colonization occurs at delivery. But before you are born, your biome communities and your immune system get instructions from your mother's flora and will be consistent with the environment provided by her. A mother who eats substances that nourish bacteria like yogurt, kefir, kombucha, and sauerkraut can be conscious that she is populating her baby's biome and providing her baby with essential nutrients to allow the immune system to develop after delivery and her influence ceases. Hormone levels are also affected by diet and biome, which are essential to the infant's brain and its developing immune system. But diet is only one contributing factor.

Before you were born, your wellbeing was also subject to maternal factors like stress, medications, allergies, and her mental state. How this happens is complex and compelling. Early life stress for the fetus can alter the *hypothalamic pituitary axis* (that part of the brain that is the conductor of the glandular orchestra which sits at the base of the brain and secretes a variety of hormones and chemicals) and the *autonomic nervous system* (responsible for your "fight-or-flight" instinct, digestion, sweating, and much more and largely responsible for later behavioral and physical changes as the child ages). Asthma and eczema, mentioned previously, are two results of this disruption, and there are likely many more.

Prenatal and early stressors in infants can affect their immune systems and their development very early and impact the rest of their lives. There are studies today geared to look at infants' "imprinting" by the early presence of microorganisms or lack thereof in their bowels. Imprinting is an older term for *epigenetic*, which means that your behaviors, environment, and other nongenetic influences can cause changes that affect the way your genes work (more on this in Chapter 8). The mother's environment is the earliest epigenetic set-point in a person's life. A recent epigenetic model of disease development predicted that early life exposures to nutritional imbalances, metals, maternal care variations, or other stressors within the environment can lead to altered expression of genes during a person's life, the basis for epigenetic changes.

Finally, the bacteria of the vaginal canal and breastfeeding are also critical to the biome and a lifelong alteration of flora in the baby's bowel. Some allergic and even autoimmune diseases as well as obesity may be more common if the baby is not vaginally born or later breastfed. For example, there is a 20 percent increase in childhood asthma when a baby is born by caesarean section. Babies are exposed to some organisms while they are in the womb, but all doctors agree that vaginal passage and subsequent breast-feeding are probably the most important early events in establishing the biome of the infant and seeding the bowel with healthy organisms. In fact, some mothers who have a caesarean birth are so acutely aware of this that they are opting for *vaginal seeding* or the transfer of vaginal flora after delivery to mouth, nose, or skin of their newborns.[2]

DR. BOB SAYS

Your biomes begin in your mother's womb and are affected by things that affect your mother and her lifestyle for better or worse. The influence of your mother's biomes continues straight through birth and are impacted greatly by the advantages of vaginal delivery and breastfeeding.

BIOMES AND YOUR BRAIN: BEHAVIOR AND BEYOND

Obviously, there is nothing you can do to return to your mother's womb. What I want you to take away from these maternal connections is how our biomes' influence extends way beyond the gut all the way to your brain. Yes, your brain. All brain cells follow the rules of the immune response genes, just like peripheral cells do, meaning that antigens and foreign materials can be accepted or rejected on the basis of something called our *histo* (tissue) compatibility (accepted or not) genes. The same things that go on in

---

[2] Many doctors feel vaginal seeding could expose their babies to dangerous bacteria like strep or staph that women can harbor after birth and is dependent on a woman's personal hygiene. If vaginal seeding is chosen, it should be done in a medical center that could test for the appropriate organisms.

the rest of your body—clearance of damaged cells, removal of unwanted intruders, and pruning nerve cells for extra efficiency—go on in your brain, only on an extraordinarily complex and controlled level.

Your brain is a very privileged immunological site with resident immune cells that protect it from infection and the products of injury. These cells depend on the immune system and the biome of the bowel to support its activities and feelings. (I suspect a bad meal can produce doom and gloom feelings because of this.) Intestinal microbes change the growth and function of those resident immune cells, while also supporting nerve cells that make your brain's connections extremely resilient and remodel certain areas after an injury like a trauma or a stroke. They are not first responders but more like dedicated electricians and technicians on call to make sure your brain is and remains intact. Consider two of the most amazing of these cells: *microglial cells* and *astrocytes*.

Microglial cells perform the functions of white cells within the brain: they are like a robotic vacuum roaming around and eating up bacteria or viruses, presenting foreign substances to antigen-presenting cells as the first line of defense within the immune system, and producing cytokines or communication molecules to invoke inflammation when it is necessary. While this is going on in the brain's "gated community," these cells are influenced directly by the bugs in your bowel and probably in other areas like your skin and reproductive zones. For example, germ-free mice have defective microglial development in their brains from birth. So, we can speculate that too much use of antibiotics early in life might adversely affect the development of these immune cells in the human brain with terrible consequences like psychiatric or behavioral issues and even a propensity to illnesses like meningitis in later life.

Astrocytes are the most abundant *glial cells* in the brain—nonneuronal (i.e., not nerve) cells that interact with microglial and other cells in the brain. Astrocytes supervise the border where spinal fluid enters and leaves your brain and maintain the integrity of the accompanying spinal fluid filtration mechanism. They monitor the brain's blood flow, facilitate nutrient transport, and regulate the excitability of neurons as a result of immune events. In doing so, astrocytes actually perform immune functions, getting information from the body's immune system so it is able to recognize bacterial and viral intruders.

But the most fascinating part of the brain's connection to your body's immune system and the biomes that inform it is the growing understanding of how they influence behavior and other diseases not normally connected to immunity.

Let us go back to diet. Much of the scientific literature deals with the effects of diets on germ-free mice (those without a biome) that I had experience with, and watching these mice gave me pause. The brains of these mice are decidedly different from the brains of mice with normal mouse diets, and I noticed that the germ-free mice were quite antisocial. (This observation was reported by others as well.) Unlike their germy peers, they preferred to stay in the recesses of their cages. But once the diet was changed and a biome developed, the mice again became social with their cagemates. Today, scientists know which probiotic organisms to add back to the mouse gut in order to allow them to socialize again. This gives me great hope that these probiotics might eventually help humans who suffer from antisocial behavior issues. It is not easy research, but the possibilities are tremendous.

Similarly, your immune system may have a major role to play in conditions like autism, schizophrenia, depression, Parkinson's, and perhaps many others. For example, children with autism have some strange biomes and unusual organisms in their stool. Interestingly, bacteria within the bowel can send signals to the *enteric nervous system* (nerve endings in the bowel) that eventually bring the brain and central nervous system into the picture.

I have always thought of autism as an immune disorder that begins at birth—rather than the completely discredited idea that it comes from vaccines—or perhaps because of an alteration of immune function later in life. I now believe it and, as we have learned more about the intimate connections of the bowel and the brain, think that the biome is one—and a major one—of many influencers of autism and other divergent behavior. There are few studies so far but in one, an organism called *Clostridia* was potentially implicated in autism: children given Vancomycin, a very potent antibiotic that is not absorbed in the intestine but can wreak havoc on the gut biome and kill many bugs like *Clostridia*, showed regression of characteristic symptoms of this autism. When the antibiotic was suspended, the children reverted to their autistic behavior.

Just as important is the likely role of biomes with regard to dementia. Researchers working with mice that had a murine version of Alzheimer's disease unexpectedly found them to have less brain pathology (clumps of protein called amyloid and neurofibrillary tangles typical of the condition) after being given huge doses of antibiotics, which killed off most of the gut bacteria in the mouse. As a result, it was entirely possible the way that organisms in the gut influenced the secretion of chemicals that control the workings of immune cells in the brain and certain organisms in the bowel of these mice actually promoted their version of dementia. There are even studies that would suggest that parasitic infestation of the gut might be useful in preventing Alzheimer's disease. Some investigators suspect that the astrocytes ApoE4 gene is an "immune protector" gene. Perhaps these astrocytes in the brain, a specific aspect of immune protection, are part of a separate neural immune system, and the ApoE4 gene is there to help them go on the attack against brain parasites in primitive societies.

The implications of this research could be that inflammation in the gut with its attendant migration of pathologic organisms could affect the brain's health and its progression to degeneration. We have no doubt that the flora of one's gut is responsible for "bad bowel diseases" like Crohn's disease, ulcerative colitis, and irritable bowel syndrome, but also disorders like autism, Parkinson's, and Alzheimer's? One can only dream of the possibilities, but you can see the essential long-term consequences of these connections.

With an aging population increasingly affected by the scourge of diseases like dementia that know no cure, we can only hope that immunity strong means as much for our mental health as our physical health in the future.

DR. BOB SAYS

Your biomes are important to things you never considered, such as vaccine efficacy and your behavior. The nervous system of the bowel and your brain connect through your biomes. In fact, disorders like autism and diseases of the central nervous system like Alzheimer's may have a direct relationship to the biome. Imagine changing behavior with food!

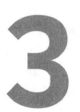

Stressing Out Your Biological Soul
The Mind-Body Connection to Immunity Strong

Like most college students trying to get into medical school, exams stressed me out. I ate poorly or nothing at all. I was in a bad mood. I was exhausted. I got so stressed I made myself sick. But I didn't connect my stress to my illness. Then I read Hans Selye's *The Stress of Life*, and for the first time, I understood just how deeply our brains and immune systems are connected.

Selye is often called the "discoverer of stress," specifically biological stress, its connection to disease, and the belief that the immune system is integrated with all physiological systems, particularly stress hormones. *The Stress of Life*, first published in 1956, was an international bestseller. While it was hardly Selye's first book or research on stress and the immune system (he was a nominee for the Nobel Prize in Physiology or Medicine in 1949), it helped his ideas gain real traction with aspiring medical students like me. Before Selye, we knew the brain was directly involved with the immune system and the recognition of foreign invaders. But Selye's idea that the hormone axis in the brain (hypothalamic gonadal, to be exact) was adversely affected by stress created whole new subspecialties—hybrid disciplines called *psychoneuroimmunology* (the study of the mind-body connection in resistance to disease) and *psycho-neuro-immuno-endocrinology* (the study the mind-body connection to immune responses, neurological processes, and endocrine functions). Those subspecialties are mouthfuls, I know, but don't stress; you don't have a spelling test or any exam in this book. But even if you did stress, thanks to Selye, you could appreciate what I did not all those years ago: that stress can make you sick.

Pressure, change, worry, uncertainty, doubt, feeling out of or lacking control, having too much or not enough responsibility—these are just some sources of stress most of us experience every day at home or at work, while commuting, trying to meet deadlines, maintaining relationships, going through a breakup or divorce, having kids, buying a house, paying for college, fighting or helping someone fight disease, making a big presentation, dealing with the loss of a loved one . . . phew, just *writing* all that stressed me out. I think it is fair to say we all understand to some degree that stress has psychological effects. But its physiological effects on your biological soul beyond, say, an anxiety attack or ulcer, are less understood. All your thoughts and thinking, not just what you do and the environment you live in, influence bodily functions, and brain-mind connections are followed by physiological responses, most notably on your immune system.

In fact, the power of the mind, the depth of belief in ourselves or a higher being, and the kindness of one's heart can evoke positive feelings that not only boost your immune system, but also might be weapons against disease. And vice versa. Recent research has explored issues of grief on immune functions. In stress, the hormones affect the cardiovascular system and also the immune system. The effects can be long-lasting in someone who has experienced loss. Of course, grief is common in our lives after a loss, but with too many people to count experiencing the incompressible and sudden loss of a loved one during the COVID-19 pandemic, the work came to the forefront. Studies cited in the *New York Times* showed that bereaved parents and spouses may "have a higher risk for cardiovascular disease, infections, cancer and chronic diseases like diabetes" and are twice as likely to die within three months of a loss than those not bereaved. Dr. Chris Fagundes, who works in psychoneuroimmunology at Rice University, has studied people who feel grief and depression and their immune systems' markers for inflammation like C-reactive protein and shifts of lymphocyte populations. Over time, he saw this can result in autoimmune disease.

Ready for more? This chapter explores how stress and resulting sleeplessness, unhappiness, depression, and isolation can weaken your biological soul and how stress reduction measures and lifestyle choices and spiritual pursuits like meditation, yoga, faith, as well as diet, exercise, social connection, sexual relations, and even just smiling, boost immunity and can strengthen it.

DR. BOB SAYS

The difference between us and an antelope running from a lion is that the antelope's stress is momentary. An antelope doesn't have time to worry, whereas we worry for long periods of time. This worry can make you sick and chronic stress can have distinct effects on your immune system.

STRESS AND SLEEP

In 2020, the *Journal of the American Medical Association* (JAMA) described a retrospective study conducted in Sweden of 2,244,193 people diagnosed with stress-related disorders like posttraumatic stress disorder (PTSD) and their connection to impaired educational performance and general cognition.[1] Besides the subjects, the study also looked at siblings of individuals with stress-related disorders and over a million age-matched controls. Among the autoimmune diseases that were found were Crohn's disease, lupus, and rheumatoid arthritis. A 2018 retrospective study published in

---

[1] Retrospective studies look at people who have a condition/disease before the study begins; prospective studies that follow people over time and before they develop symptoms.

JAMA showed an increased risk for developing autoimmune disease in people suffering from PTSD. Before these prominent studies, several smaller studies offered proof that the immune system was directly affected by stress but nothing of this scale. The connection most likely happens through your body's chemical messengers and mediators that are hormones. Levels of hormones in the blood, particularly corticosteroid hormones, change with stress and are the likely agents of change and gene expression during stressful events, but sex hormones might also be involved. The data are convincing.

That said, I and many others have believed this intuitively for decades. Most of us will never suffer from PTSD, but experienced early in life, stress can cause long-lasting changes in physiology and behavior. Stress lowers our immune system's resistance and opens us up to various infections through immunosuppression, specifically through increased corticosteroids, which are potent immunosuppressants. The biological reason for this immunosuppression is the influence of the nervous and endocrine systems on the immune system that leads to inflammation, a condition that results in pain, fever, redness, and feelings of being unwell accompanied by loss of appetite, excessive fatigue, and/or sleeplessness (more on inflammation in Chapter 6).

Of those things, lack of sleep can be most devastating to your mind and biological soul. Data going back decades have shown that sleep is critical to good health. But it is only more recently that stress has been associated with lack of sleep and that it affects your memory and mood as well. When it comes to immunity, we now know lack of sleep enhances immune-mediated inflammatory diseases and that the sleep cycle is of particular importance to proper immune homeostasis. Resistance to infection is also a major aspect of the lack of sleep. All this knowledge about stress, immunity, and sleep is a big part of the reason why training of doctors now incorporates rest and sleep during internships and residencies: Many studies showed that a lack of sleep encouraged errors and increased the amount of time that trainees were sick and unable to work.

Some scientists have even described a "feed forward loop" involving poor sleep quality that can affect inflammatory responses and even antiviral immunity. For example, Dr. Michael Irwin, Director of Mindful Awareness at UCLA's Cousins Center for Psychoneuroimmunology, notes that circadian rhythms are critical aspects of the sleep mechanism and essential to control inflammation and the antiviral immune response. Specifically, lack of sleep impacted all measures of inflammation routinely measured in Dr. Irwin's clinic and my own (TNF, interleukin 6, and C-reactive protein levels in the blood) to determine degrees of inflammation.

In my early years of research, I did experiments with light and dark and bacterial resistance. Mice kept in cages and never exposed to light had difficulty warding off bacterial infections and died quickly when challenged, whereas the mice kept in the light and dark cycles had no problems. These early experiments suggested that the circadian rhythms of the body (the light-dark cycles), had a lot to do with regulation of the immune system with ramifications for those of us who are light deprived. It's not just seasonal affective disorder, but also the lack of sunlight that impairs this immunity. The rhythmic changes that occur with the light-dark cycle involve the pituitary and the internal secretion of melatonin. And that brings us back to mind-body and immunity: both your innate and adaptive immunity depend on your circadian rhythm.

Your spleen (the Alcatraz of your body) has cells within it that are regulated by circadian rhythms. Moreover, CD4 T cells show circadian variations in the production of cytokines, those essential communication molecules (specifically, IL-2, interferon gamma, and IL-4). It is likely rheumatoid patients have stiffness in the morning and lupus patients tend to have flares of their disease when the seasons change due to the circadian rhythms and the change of the light-dark cycles; hormones within the body respond to light and darkness, and in turn, affect immune functions. In addition, studies in Scandinavian countries, where light is at a premium in the winter months, have shown vitamin D (which we get from sunlight and food) plays a role in lowered infection resistance of humans not exposed to light. Since vitamin D deficiency is very common, many medical professionals recommend vitamin D supplements even when they don't recommend other supplements.

But neither vitamin D nor any food or supplements, or even a solid sleep routine alone, can overcome stress.

DR. BOB SAYS

Stress affects sleep and sleep is essential for homeostasis, a balanced and stable internal state, and being immunity strong. Lack of sleep and a disturbance of the light-dark cycles in the brain can affect immune functions, as both your adaptive and innate immunity depend on your circadian rhythm.

DE-STRESS YOUR BIOLOGICAL SOUL: MEDITATION, YOGA, ACUPUNCTURE, AND EXERCISE

The truth is, anything that relaxes you has its benefits. But there is hard evidence the following activities, all of which can be performed in public or private (unlike sex, which we will consider next), connect to immunity strong:

- Meditation, Tai Chi, and Qigong
- Acupuncture
- Yoga
- Exercise

Meditation, Tai Chi, and Qigong

Dr. Lucas G. Irwin is a big supporter of mindfulness meditation, as am I. Mindfulness meditation focuses your attention and decreases your reactivity to stressful stimuli. This relaxation response enhances the tone of the *vagus nerve*. The vagus nerve carries signals from the brain to the heart, lungs, digestive system, and other organs, and vice versa. One of its novel functions is controlling the inflammatory response through suppressing the activity of proinflammatory cytokines through the *cholinergic anti-inflammatory pathway*. It also diminishes the response of the *hypothalamic pituitary adrenal axis*— the same axis that Selye discussed—which is the reason you have elevated cortisol and adrenaline during stressful events.

Irwin found the amount of meditation practiced in a six-week compassion meditation program correlated with the decrease in one cytokine called *interleukin 6* (IL-6), a proinflammatory cytokine with stimulant activity (which, for example, elevated in COVID-19). Investigators studying the relaxation response have also found that the meditation had a positive effect on the immune system, which many psychoneuroimmunologists refer to as a sensory system unto itself.

If sitting still and meditating is not for you, try Tai Chi or Qigong. Of the two, Qigong (pronounced chee-gong) is probably the less familiar to most people in the Western world. Qigong translates to "energy work" and is like a millennia-old Chinese form of yoga that coordinates body-posture and movement, breathing, and meditation to open the flow of energy through the body. Tai Chi is an ancient Chinese martial art but little of its forms have anything to do with self-defense, only postures and motions that are sometimes called "shadowboxing" and "meditation in motion." Like Qigong, it is usually practiced in groups in parks and other locations across the country. I was pretty late to the game when I first encountered it in Shanghai in 2007 while helping with a medical conference. I was staying in the legendary Peace Hotel, and my room faced the famous Bund waterfront area along the Huangpu River. Every morning, dozens of people gathered and moved in unison for 30 minutes or so. When I asked why, they said it was their way of meditating and staying healthy. These forms of Tai Chi are all about the yin and yang or the light and dark balance of the internal and external and the physical and spiritual world. Tai Chi and Qigong are often practiced in groups.

While there are no fixed protocols to teach people how to use Tai Chi and Qigong as a movement-based mind-body therapies, Tai Chi and Qigong have been linked for centuries to reduced stress, homeostasis, and immunity through controlling breathing and a sense of wellbeing through movement. Today, there are studies that demonstrate how they have a positive impact on immune system functioning and inflammatory processes. Early papers from China suggested that inflammatory markers like the C-reactive proteins and some populations of immune cells decreased with the practice of Qigong. (The Chinese indicate that innate immune cells increased compared to normal controls; there was no effect on natural killer T cells or dendritic cells.) A more definitive 2020 review in the journal *Medicine* indicated, by meta-analysis or the review of many studies from China and other parts of the world, that Tai Chi and Qigong are capable of modulating the immune system and the inflammatory biomarker responses. It takes roughly four weeks of practice with an expert and the data suggests that both the innate and adaptive immune responses are enhanced, and the biomarkers for inflammation are lowered. In addition, two studies have indicated that after 12 weeks on a controlled series of experiments involving Qigong, gene expression as demonstrated by the molecular NF-kB signal pathways was altered. This molecular pathway altered the number of secreted cytokines (those communication molecules of your immune system) particularly the proinflammatory ones—so much so that the studies recommended Tai Chi and Qigong for those infected with viruses like COVID-19.

To my mind, all these forms are again where the rubber hits the road regarding the biological soul. The capacity of the human mind is an intrinsic and changeable aspect of mindfulness. This mindfulness is an awareness that emerges through paying attention nonjudgmentally to the unfolding experience around you and us moment by moment—to your purpose in the present moment. Sounds heavy, and it is. Making this important connection to being mindful of the stress that surrounds and impacts your biological soul is a major link to your longevity.

Acupuncture

As a visiting professor in China in 1989, I met two kinds of doctors: those who practiced orthodox medicine and those who practiced traditional Chinese medicine, which dates back 8,000 years, including acupuncture (the practice of inserting needles into the body to reduce pain or induce anesthesia) and moxibustion (acupuncture with burning herbs placed on top of the acupuncture needles). The traditional Chinese medicine doctors considered acupuncture and moxibustion major ways to boost immune function and decrease inflammation and used them to control allergy, infections, and autoimmunity. I will never forget visiting the People's Liberation Army's General Hospital's Moxibustion Clinic in Beijing and seeing clouds of smoke from all the burning herbs. I found the doctors in modern hospitals who practiced this traditional Chinese medicine fascinating.

Acupuncture has since gained a foothold in modern-day medicine in the West. The theory of acupuncture centers around something called qi energy or the energy that flows through the body's energy pathways known as meridians. Chinese medicine believes that disease is caused by an imbalance of the flow of this energy. Thus, acupuncture targets 350 to 400 points where needles can be placed in the body to restore that energy. Practitioners and physicians use different acupoints, and different times of application, making it difficult to acquire standardized immunological data, but since acupuncture is used to control pain and inflammation, there must be some effect on immunity.

Most scientists believe that acupuncture leads to the secretion of endorphins or pain modifiers within the body. There is one study in which a form of bacterial arthritis induced in rats was modified with acupuncture. The study also said that monocyte or macrophage cells of innate immunity and the T cells of innate and adaptive immunity were affected by the manual placement of the needles. Imagine if someday this could lead to a link to a cure for diseases like rheumatoid arthritis. There is no definitive immunological data to support these claims, but even without it, acupuncture has become a standard in the West and is now offered as an optional course for attending physicians at most hospitals. The procedure is also covered by many major insurance companies.

Yoga

The 5000-year-old discipline of yoga teaches mindfulness, improves our wellness, and has extreme benefits for us through the immune system. First of all, the very root of the word yoga comes from the Sanskrit word for join or unite and uniting mind, spirit, and all aspects of yourself is essential to destressing. Specifically, I am talking about a broader connection to spirituality or concern with your soul and those of others (as opposed to material things), which is beneficial to immune protection because it offers you peace. This spiritual peace has no relationship to which God you worship, religion you choose, or if you believe or worship at all. In *Molecules of Emotion: Why You Feel the Way You Feel* (1997), Dr. Candace Pert, a neuroscientist who is known as "the Mother of Psychoneuroimmunology," called this peace "freedom from disturbance" and "better vibration"—a "spark of oneness [that] increases the number of endorphins in the body." I call endorphins the feel-good molecules of the immune system, because they help give you peace and put you in a blissful state of balance.

My wife, Carolyn, is my go-to expert for all things spiritual. She likes to say that we are a community of animals and the good and evil within our bodies are in a constant fight for this balance. I get it now. When these competing emotions in concert with the immune system are in balance, they can naturally overcome disease and encourage a homeostatic state. And remarkably, the immune system maintains this homeostasis thousands of times daily in an imperceptible manner. Yoga can help your immune system do it even better.

There are many branches of yoga—from extreme to those involving beer and goats (separately, mind you)—but the most popular in the Western world is hatha yoga, which uses a set of exercises or postures to align all parts of your body, manipulate respiration, and create balance of strength and flexibility. Yoga has also been shown to assist bone growth and act as an antidepressant. The relief of stress through yoga, like in Tai Chi and Qigong, also has been shown to have direct effects on cytokine production. Most important for your immune system, however, is that yoga increases the levels of *superoxide dismutase* (an enzyme that changes oxygen radicals into plain oxygen) and *glutathione* (an antioxidant produced in your cells) that are major defenses against oxidative stress, which can damage cells and contribute to aging.

Perhaps most intriguing for the future, a neuro-immune study found that yoga positively affects gene expression profiles in immune cells. This could be epigenetics at its best: a behavioral practice that influences gene expression (more on this in Chapter 8). Gene expression differences were found in peripheral blood mononuclear cells of those who practice yoga. In another study, mind-body interventions lowered the production of a chemical substance called NF-kB, which alters the levels of cytokines and helps to alleviate stress. As Dr. Ivana Buric of Coventry University in the United Kingdom said in *Frontiers of Immunology* (2017), "These activities are leaving what we would call a molecular signature in our cells that reverses the effect stress or anxiety would have on the body by changing how our genes are expressed."

Exercise

I ran the NYC marathon in 1984. I trained tirelessly in the months and weeks leading up to it. Sure, I was elated about the challenge, but I was exhausted. I developed a dry cough and got little sleep. My muscles ached around the clock. I had blackened toes, dehydration, and an urge to eat everything in sight. At the time, I wondered if my elevated exercise regimen had any beneficial effect on my immune system. I seemed to be experiencing the opposite. The short answer was no.

Moderate exercise strengthens your immune system. It results in a rise of white cells and a redistribution of cells between the blood compartment and the lymph nodes and other peripheral tissues in organs like the liver, lung, and kidney. But recent research has shown that prolonged periods of *intensive* exercise like

I was doing while training are not necessarily good for you and can depress immunity. That's right, the profound stress induced with extreme athletic activities can be a downer from a biological perspective. In other words, don't stress yourself out doing something that is supposed to help you not stress out!

Prolonged exercise may impair T cell responses, natural killer cells, and white cell functions. Cytokine balances are also changed with prolonged stressful exercises and immune responses to primary antigen exposure. This may lead to alterations in what we called mucosal immunity and why the elite runners frequently talk about symptoms associated with upper respiratory tract infections during periods of heavy training and competition. Mucosal immunity, or the immunity around the mouth, nose, vagina, rectum, and the entirety of the GI tract, is the border patrol of your biological soul. Mucosal immunity even has its own immunoglobulin or antibody class called *secretory IgA* and intense periods of exercise lower secretory IgA antibodies.

Single short bouts of what I call feel-good exercise, however, result in endorphin release. What I mean by this is a workout that gets your heart rate up but is not super stressful—nothing that pushes your body to its limits of endurance, especially when you have not been exercising regularly. This kind of aerobic exercise like swimming, running three to six miles per day, or just walking for one to two miles daily can improve immunity through reductions of inflammation, maintenance of thymus gland size (when you are younger), and alteration in the composition of older versus younger immune cells. It also enhances immune surveillance or the process by which your immune system cells identify, monitor and destroy infected, cancerous, or precancerous cells, which is essential to our understanding of aging and the decline of immune function.

Psychological stress in people who exercise is also ameliorated for reasons that are not totally clear, but probably as a result of mindfulness that I spoke of previously and those endorphins that provide feelings of pleasure. It's a kind of mobile meditation that most runners know as a "runner's high." The important thing to understand is that extreme is bad, especially as we age. Of course, the individual has to have enough energy and health to embark on such an exercise program. Older individuals, patients living with cancer, people those with chronic viral infections such as HIV and COVID-19, and obese people would be better off and benefit more from small exercise events that build into more moderate programs.

DR. BOB SAYS

Mindful meditation, yoga, acupuncture, and exercise—but not extreme exercise—are three ways to reduce stress and enrich your immune response. Stress is a source of immunosuppression. Inflammation from injury, psychological or physical, can alter immune resistance through defined mechanisms that include the brain, glands and hormones, and the immune system.

SEX AND SOCIALIZATION

People ask me about sex and the immune system all the time, wanting to know if it's good for their bodies or if sex is beneficial to the immune system. I must admit the first thing that pops into my head is "The Pickle Gambit" episode of Larry David's *Curb Your Enthusiasm*. In the episode, Larry's friend's golden-child nephew breaks his elbow in a freak pickle jar accident, which prevents him from masturbating and relaxing, which in turn turns him into a monster. Larry's solution is to hire a prostitute he knows, because he needs some release from all that stress. Whether you find the scene amusing, disturbing, or both, Larry's premise is spot on: Sex and sexual release (orgasm) are some of the most relaxing activities that one can enjoy. It isn't just sex, however; hugging one another, petting a cat or dog, and strong relationships and socialization affect homeostasis because they de-stress us. But let's talk about sex first.

There is plenty of evidence going back decades that having sex affects all aspects of human life and a vigorous sex life is good for your biological soul. People who have had more sex (without resulting in sexually transmitted diseases or viruses) have more mucosal IgA antibody and fewer sick days at work. One prospective study followed college students into adulthood and showed that sexual intercourse and even masturbation enhanced the health of both men and women. In addition, sexually active women in one study had less cardiac events later in life. Sexual arousal and orgasm also induce an increase in what are called sympathetic activities of the nervous system as well as the enhancement of *catecholamine*, a hormone made by your adrenal glands that acts as a neurotransmitter and helps you respond to stress, as well as increasing amounts of the hormone *prolactin*, an immune stimulant from the pituitary gland in blood plasma.[2]

In a 2004 study called "Effects of Sexual Arousal on Lymphocyte Subset Circulation and Cytokine Production in Man," published in *Neuroimmunomodulation*, the effects of masturbation-induced orgasm on lymphocyte circulation and cytokine production were studied in young men. White cell and lymphocyte subsets were analyzed via a method called flow cytometry in which the cells could be labeled with certain kinds of markers and the types of cells like lymphocytes measured. The study was exceedingly small, but the results were startling in that they noted a transient increase in adrenaline and prolactin because of the orgasm, which resulted in an increase in the number of white cells, in particular natural killer cells which are very potent antiviral lymphocytes. In contrast, the T cell and B cell subpopulations as well as the production of interleukins and tumor necrosis factor alpha were unaffected by the sexual activity. These findings, at

---

[2] Abnormally high amounts of prolactin have been reported by me and others as a cause of autoimmune disease in some patients. Rarely, I do see patients that have microtumors in their pituitary glands and produce super amounts of this hormone and consequential immune disease. But there is nothing abnormal in the amounts of prolactin produced during normal sexual activity.

least in males, indicate that components of the innate immune system are activated by sexual arousal and orgasm.

Another interesting aspect of sexual relations is that this activity actually causes immune system changes in women that increase the chances of conception. As we covered briefly in Chapter 1 and will cover in more detail in Chapter 9, a woman's immune function changes during pregnancy and after childbirth. However, the immune response also changes during and across the menstrual cycle. I was always intrigued by this since I could ask patients with rheumatoid arthritis about the relationship of their period to the pain and discomfort of their disease and they would always tell me where they were in regard to their menstrual cycle. Now investigators at Indiana University have shown that sexual cycles play a major role in these immune changes, the likes of which are also found in women who are sexually active versus those who are sexually abstinent.

The investigators reported that sexually active women experience greater changes in the proteins that T cells use to communicate, namely cytokines and chemokines from helper T cells. Higher levels of TH1 T cells were also found in these women during what we call the follicular phase of the menstrual cycle, a period when the ovary follicles are maturing (eggs that mother drops to be fertilized by sperm.) Antibody levels were also different in both groups (sexually active versus sexually inactive) of women. Secretory antibodies, like IgA, are typically found in the mucus of the female reproductive tract and these antibodies are found in the mouth and in the intestine and just about anywhere where there are mucous membranes. Because of this, they can interfere with the movement of sperm and other aspects of fertilization. Investigators hypothesized that they were really looking at an immune system that was readying the woman's uterus for the possibility of pregnancy just as a result of sexual activity. All of this would indicate that the immune system is extremely active in the process of fertilization as well as pregnancy.

I have interviewed many women who have been infertile for reasons that were associated with stress, long after multiple fertility studies were completed. After resolution of that stress through psychotherapy or through appropriate drug use to combat the stress, they would suddenly become pregnant, which is something far fewer women were doing globally during the recent global pandemic. The birth rate during the pandemic was the lowest observed since 1973, with hundreds of thousands of fewer births reported in the United States. Many countries are reporting similar declines, including China, which expected a decline of more than 10 percent, and Italy, which expected a decline of more than 21 percent. Demographers and economists rightly worry about this baby bust and whether it is temporary. I worry about whether it might also say something about the pandemic increasing our isolation and desocialization. COVID-19 limited our ability to socialize the way we had before for more than a year for most of us.

Levels of stress leading to depression and suicidality increased by double digits during the pandemic. According to the COVID Impact Survey by NORC at the University of Chicago, approximately two-thirds of Americans surveyed said they felt depressed and lonely or hopeless once during the previous week during the pandemic and almost 20 percent felt that way more than three times. Data from prisons and many long-term care facilities where people were isolated reveal major issues revolving around a lack of activity.

Simply put, isolation or the lack of socialization is not healthy for anyone. Like prisoners in solitary confinement, it can lead to depression and lowered host resistance at any age. This was a major topic of discussion and concern about children not being able to socialize with friends and being kept from their classmates for most if not all of a school year and longer because of the pandemic shutdown and worry about spreading the virus. The effects on their mental and physical health are only just beginning to be understood.

For seniors, the effects of isolation were of particular concern during the pandemic as well but were well understood long before. Getting old is stressful, and immunosenescence is inevitable as we do, but our biological soul wants to try and keep us living long lives. Isolation, and by extension loneliness, is affecting its purpose deeply. "Social Isolation and Loneliness in Older Adults," a 2020 study from the National Academies of Sciences, Engineering, and Medicine, linked both conditions to serious health conditions like dementia and premature death from all causes that could be as harmful as smoking, obesity, and a lack of physical activity.

During the pandemic of 2020, we heard of people buying enormous amounts of gym equipment to maintain their physical activity, but they still missed the camaraderie of gyms, even if just to have people around them. Perhaps this adds an explanation for the success of Peloton bikes and other exercise equipment that links us to trainers and group classes. But you don't need to drop thousands on fancy equipment to get the same benefits. If you need a boost, get out there and meet someone and take a walk together. Not a people person? How about a pet? Pet owners have decreased blood pressure and lower cholesterol, and the presence of pets increases immune resistance and enhances homeostasis. Oxytocin is released when you hug a pet, or for that matter, when you hug a human being. Called the "love hormone"—because it shows itself in high concentration after love making, hugging, and kissing—oxytocin is actually part hormone and part essential protein and comes from the pituitary gland at base of the brain, where the brain-body connection likely begins.

Oxytocin has salutary effects on the immune system and could be a major connection between the brain and immunity. When you're stressed, oxytocin can remove the effects of cortisone and increase your resistance to infection. It can rebalance your system. It might even stimulate the production of cytokines.[3] Oxytocin also has a major role in the development of your thymus gland (your immune system's city hall), the bone marrow where large numbers of lymphocytes are formed, and the overall integrity of immune functions and maintenance of the immune system. This

---

[3] Oxytocin nerve cells at the base of the brain can produce some of these cytokines and other inflammatory molecules in the brains of rats, and I have a hunch that the same process is operating in humans.

could be the way the immune system gets perked up after a hug and even more during sexual relations. So, you see the need to love someone or something like a pet runs deep when it comes to immunity strong. It all comes back to love or at least kindness—both to your biological soul and others.

I hope you now realize that the integration of the immune system with the brain is a major aspect of the biological soul and immunity strong. The immune system is ravaged by the stresses of life. Longevity ends when we consider the things that we do to ourselves, our inability to relax, exercise, and move on with life in a healthy way. And here is an easy way to get started on the path to immunity strong: Turn that frown upside down. A growing number of researchers and studies show smiling, and by extension laughter and optimism, are simple and powerful ways to boost your immune system and resist infection by increasing your immune cells and antibodies. One study even showed increased natural killer T cell activity in males who were watching a funny movie as compared to a group watching a neutral movie, in which they saw no such response. The evidence might still be growing but nothing about it will hurt you. In fact, smiling uses fewer muscles than frowning and laughter is contagious—one of the few contagions this immunologist recommends!

DR. BOB SAYS

A lot of good things happen because of sexual activity, but the fact that your immune system is enhanced is not the first to come to mind. That's right: Sexual relations and all socialization is essential to immunity. But you don't need to have sex to have these benefits: Relationships with others (or even a pet) have the same effect as making love. What this means is "love" is the winner here and essential to the health of your biological soul.

The Most Wanted List
More on Viruses, Bacteria, and Parasites

For decades, the FBI has maintained a list of its ten most wanted fugitives—criminals who have done terrible things and have eluded capture, sometimes for years. In the FBI headquarters of your biological soul, some of the most wanted criminals that cause diseases like multiple sclerosis, rheumatoid arthritis, and lupus are unknown and, as of now, cannot be prevented with vaccines. Many of the rest are antigens—viruses, bacteria, and parasites—and they have been and are doing terrible things to us. Like the real FBI's Most Wanted, some of these criminals have been caught (polio, smallpox, measles) and others (COVID-19, influenza) have had their ongoing damage mitigated by vaccines and therapies. But many antigens have eluded capture and remain on our immune system's most wanted list—untreatable and deadly.

Like real criminals, these antigens all act differently. Some attack violently, quickly overwhelming the immune system and making it incapable of a defensive response. Others are like con artists and confidence men—masters of disguise or "opportunistic infections"—that can trick our immune systems and evolve to avoid our defenses to reproduce, as we all learned when the COVID-19 variants from Britain, Brazil, South Africa, New York, and India appeared.

As we learned in Chapter 1, your immune system's first responders provide two sophisticated types of protections—innate and adaptive response—that succeed far more than they fail when it comes to fighting crime. Your innate response is your first line of defense and efficiently catches and prosecutes antigenic criminals better than the actual FBI or any police department ever could. It is an ancient component of your immune system that relies on those proteins known as pattern recognition receptors (alarmins and defensins) and other signals dependent on receptors to defend you against common criminals and dispatch them 24/7 without you ever knowing. But our innate response only knows how to sort criminals into two groups: something that belongs in your body's city (self) and something external affecting it (nonself). When the criminals are too difficult for your innate first responders to handle, they sound the alarm for more help and your adaptive response team arrives to determine whether or not further action is needed.

This chapter tells a fuller story of what happens next—when "most wanted" antigens like COVID-19 or HIV overwhelm all our first responders and your immune system fails. What happens when these viruses and others go undetected by our innate response? How are they so good at hiding? As in all things with our immune system, there is strength in knowledge and understanding, not just action, when it comes to these questions and the biological soul's most wanted. After all, most scientists believe that it is only a matter of time before another novel "most wanted" virus wreaks havoc again.

DR. BOB SAYS

Many diseases that plague humans, like rheumatoid arthritis, lupus, multiple sclerosis, and vasculitis do not have known causes. Doctors have clues on those causes from criminals like

COVID-19 or organisms like streptococcus. Your immune system's detectives use these same clues to remember criminals in its biological database.

ELUSIVE VIRUSES

Viruses make up the bulk of our "most wanted" list. They have been around since animals and plants appeared on the planet, and that's where my interest in them started as well, in plants specifically. As a young man, I was fascinated by the work of a young plant pathologist, Professor Wendel Stanley, whose early electron photos of the tobacco mosaic virus showed how it used tobacco plants to replicate. He had electron micrographic photos of the virus as crystals (they are too small for the standard microscope) and, since living things do not crystalize, confirmed that viruses cannot live independently. That's right: Viruses are not alive and cannot reproduce on their own. They use us, as well as plants and animals, for reproduction, using the cell's machinery to replicate indefinitely in every living thing on the planet. In other words, they commit their crimes and then seek to move on to other victims. And these viruses are very efficient and often sneaky criminals.

Viruses often lay in wait and assault your immune system long after they invade your body. The two I will focus on here—COVID-19 and HIV—get inside by developing an affinity for your receptors or a stickiness in your cells that is present for something else. For example, COVID-19 uses the *angiotensin converting enzyme 2* or ACE2 receptor on the cells of your lung, heart, kidney, and especially mouth, nose, and eyes. ACE2 is a receptor for control of blood pressure. It should have nothing to do with viral replication. But COVID-19 latched onto it, and by trial and error or just divine attraction, used it to enter the body.

Where COVID-19 specifically originated or whether it came from a bat, some other creature, or a laboratory is less important for you to understand than the fact that there are 150 or more unknown viruses that do not infect humans yet but exist in the animal kingdom. What is more important for you to understand is what criminals like these do to you when they jump species and get inside you like others before them. These viruses have evolved the ability to hide within our cells until, like a psychosocial stressor setting off a serial killer, some charge or spark sets it off like the fever blister or shingles rash of the well-known family of herpes viruses. Once an infection is established, the virus surfaces, knowing that our immune systems, surprised by the invasion, will vehemently and mercilessly attack it. At the beginning of most of these infections, our immune system goes through a series of convulsions—actions that indicate an assault is in progress that may signal its demise. *Autoantibodies* (immune proteins that attack your tissues and organs) develop. Cells like lymphocytes are broadly stimulated, and antibodies develop against many self-antigens (which the healthy immune system usually tolerates). The innate immune system can be confused and overwhelmed during this virus infection and the one thing that it is known for, "distinguishing self from nonself," may temporarily disappear producing autoantibodies and self-directed cells as we see in many acute infections.

But remember: Viruses don't want to kill us as hosts; they want to evade the immune system, replicate, and move on to other hosts. In the confusion, it's our first responders, as we learned in Chapter 1, that might kill us when fighting back, stopping the virus from spreading but also putting an end to us in the process. No, this is not when I tell you that what happens next makes the plot of most zombie movies not so farfetched. They are. When the host dies, the virus dies in us. But it remains "at large" in others. Those that continue to avoid capture or have their effects mitigated are our biological soul's most wanted criminals.

Infections from these viruses are exceedingly difficult to manage, and new virus infections pose challenges that are tricky; new syndromes appear like immunodeficiency in the case of HIV or an odd very bad pneumonia in the case of COVID-19. Moreover, viruses like COVID-19 have shown an ability to create variants and "upward" mutations or what is called *convergent evolution* so they can resist capture and live on within us and infect more hosts.

DR. BOB SAYS

Viruses are not alive but thrive by entering your body in curious ways and using it as reservoirs of infection. They can appear and disappear in the stealthiest manner and, like herpes infections, surface at random times.

I am sure that you are trying to get your head around all I just said as much as I still am. I spent many years of my life trying to understand the immunology of viruses as a microbiologist. Today, I spend most of my time with immunologic diseases, holding out hope that organisms like viruses are at the core and indeed the cause of our most mysterious illness and autoimmune diseases like multiple sclerosis, lupus, rheumatoid arthritis, and diabetes. My belief comes from my work with some of the most wanted like COVID-19, the symptoms from which often mimic those diseases and others we desperately need to solve like dementia. Other conditions associated with infections like chronic fatigue syndrome and fibromyalgia are also enigmas because their causes are unknown, they occur without warning, and they are difficult to treat (more on this in Chapter 10).

So, could COVID-19 and HIV offer clues to the causes of our most expensive, painful and deadly illnesses? Elusive, mysterious, and lethal, they were both difficult to diagnose and understood only after they committed mass murder. But perhaps to catch a criminal, we need to get inside the "mind" of other criminals. If there is any positive aspect of a pandemic, especially for modern medicine, it is that a viral infection that causes signs and symptoms of diseases that we know how to treat may enhance our understanding of those diseases going forward. But what a price to pay.

HIV AND COVID-19

I was there at the beginning of both HIV and COVID-19. Well, not the very beginning. As with most viruses, the origins of HIV remain unclear, though it has been traced to Central Africa in the early twentieth century when it jumped species from chimpanzees to humans. The earliest record of someone dying from HIV was in 1959 in what was then known as the Belgian Congo. Since then, it has killed 35 million people with its peak death and destruction coming in the late 1970s through the 1990s, when it secured a position as one of our "most wanted" criminals. That's where I came in.

In 1978, as a fellow in training at Rockefeller University, a colleague and I were asked to go to Memorial Sloan Kettering Hospital to draw blood from young men (they were all men) with some unfamiliar immunodeficiency. We brought the samples back to our lab to do mixed lymphocyte stimulation to see if the functions of their T cells (products of one of your embryonic stem cells that give rise to all other T cells in the body) were debilitated as the overall numbers of such cells (CD4 positive cells) seemed low in these men. Since we had no knowledge of the specific cells involved, we looked at the responses of T cells as a whole. We also had no idea that we were confronting a viral infection or that the men all identified as homosexual. This was well before the time when people would not even go into rooms accommodated by HIV-infected patients! We did not wear gloves and mouth-pipetted blood from the patients to line our dishes with cells. The sera and our tongues had only a small piece of cotton between them. Once a virus was established as the cause of the immunodeficiency, we wondered for some time if our aseptic ways were sufficient to protect us and were lucky that HIV, unlike a respiratory virus, was not transmitted through respiratory droplets but certain bodily fluids like blood, semen, breast milk, and vaginal fluids.

Like I said, we were incredibly lucky, because if we had been infected, HIV takes advantage of the immune system in many ways and is ingenious and resourceful in its attack. Unlike COVID-19, which attaches itself to receptors within selected parts of the body, we found that out later that the HIV virus uses the CD receptors (*cluster determinants* that identify certain subpopulations of T cells that make the immune system function) on your CD4 T lymphocytes or T cells to get inside.

To refresh your memory of their role as first responders, your T cells are essential to the regulation of both the innate and adaptive immune processes. It is vital to basic immune response to know which foreign substances are criminals, what they have done, and what needs to be done to step up and attack. The link to immunogenetics or what your immune system considers a criminal is the T cell CD receptor. The CD markers that your doctor talks about are like the numbers you see on the roofs of buses or police cars from a drone or a helicopter: They are identifiers for your immune system and very important to you, the host. Broadly speaking, these CD receptors are either helpers or suppressors of immune function: CD4 T cells are generally helpers and CD8 T cells are generally suppressors. The CD4 receptor on helper T cells recognizes foreign or self-proteins bound to communication molecules, and if appropriate, sparks activation of B cells and macrophages. This process is very selective and links to something called your *major histocompatibility locus* on chromosome 6, which rules your immune system. So, imagine what would happen if your CD4 T cells were dysfunctional and obliterated by a virus: Your immune system's ruler would be deposed! This is what happens with an HIV infection: There is no longer a biological soul. There is no immunity strong.

With the infected T cell population decimated, insurrections and random criminal events in HIV patients go unchecked. Patients die from otherwise harmless bacteria like those found in rice, the soil, and bread mold. They are felled by innocuous bugs from the skin or bowel or a common virus or bacteria because immunity is crippled—their true protectors and the organization of your body's first responders is gone. Meanwhile, the CD8 suppressor T cells (totally different from the CD4 helper cells) were left to fend for themselves and confused the immune system even more. CD8 T cells (suppressors in character) also recognize viral antigens, especially those that are made in the cytoplasm or nonnuclear portion of a cell. With the loss of CD4 T helper cells, however, the immune system collapses in disarray.

Don't worry, there's no test on this later. All you need to know is that there is a link between the genetics of immunity and your cellular response. HIV infected the CD4 helper cells through their receptors and obliterated them by essentially tricking some immune systems to replace the T cells that would fight off HIV with those infected by HIV.

DR. BOB SAYS

For the most part we live in near symbiosis with viruses. This is not the case with viruses like HIV and COVID-19. They decimate the immune system by being novel agents or viruses that dig into the fabric of the immune system to make your T cells dysfunctional and are usually deadly until a vaccine or therapy is developed.

Being there at the start of the HIV pandemic (the World Health Organization officially calls it an epidemic, but I and many others disagree) was horrible, novel, and unfathomable all at the same time. Adding to the horror was how HIV stigmatized gay men and IV drug users, who were most prominently infected. Hemophiliacs who required blood products were just as susceptible to the virus and the stigma, suspected of being gay or drug users when infected whether they were or not. Soon, many unsuspecting people were stigmatized and infected either through drug use, blood transfusion, and sexual contact (not just homosexual). HIV also took hold in underdeveloped countries, where heterosexual couples gave it to each other and their children. Although a vaccine was investigated, the world has developed several chemical means of treating and mitigating the effects of HIV that seems to have slowed the urgency for one. The stigma has also been reduced by celebrities like Magic Johnson, who helped educate others and dispel a few misconceptions. But that does not mean HIV has fallen off the most wanted list. It remains a very damaging virus today and affects rich and poor countries.

Unlike HIV, COVID-19 never had any stigma as it became a global pandemic because it is nonselective; it infects any person that it can enter and as a result has been deadly far quicker. COVID-19 is a respiratory virus (coronaviruses are in the "common cold" family), meaning it wreaks havoc in the lung most commonly and respiratory failure is the worst outcome. Moreover, the entire immune system is involved in the pathologic features associated with this illness. Usually, the lungs fill with fluid and then inflammatory liquid (pus). If the patient is truly unlucky, the virus produces micro clots in the lung and then a cytokine storm leading to the acute respiratory distress syndrome or ARDS I described in Greg in Chapter 1: When the lungs fail, the patient goes on an endotracheal tube and ventilator to give the patient oxygen, hoping that the immune system will balance and calm itself and the virus will cease replicating. In the first year of COVID-19, only 50 percent of people who had the tube placed in their tracheas and were artificially ventilated survived.

The curious thing about COVID-19 is that it does not attack everyone the same way. Some are asymptomatic. Most of those who are not report some kind of exhaustion. But after that? While millions have been hospitalized, millions more get only mild cold symptoms. In between them are millions more who had something like a bad flu. Some people lose their taste and smell; others retain all their senses. Unlike viruses like measles or influenza, young people are mostly unaffected but for those over age 65 and those with comorbidities like heart or lung disease, it can be devastating. We suspect these differences are because everyone's immune system is specific to that person and his or her family. But that does not mean one has immunity for the future. As noted at the start of this chapter, over time, viruses like COVID-19 and influenza become endemic and mutate. The immune system will be baffled again and need help with antiviral drugs or strong immunosuppressants until there is a new or existing vaccine to at least mitigate the effects, as there are almost no medications that will be effective. Hundreds of millions of people died worldwide from the COVID-19 pandemic before the vaccines were administered. But even with those in hand, we must be vigilant, especially for the variants—some of which are more transmissible and deadly.

Viruses like COVID-19 are like a bad gift that keeps on giving, making us protect ourselves every year with new vaccines against mutant variants. And no matter what you've read, vaccines are essential in helping our first responders combat viruses and do far better for us than bad. Vaccines may eventually eliminate common viruses like herpes zoster infection or shingles, a neurotrophic virus or one that resides quietly in nerve cells until activated by stress or diseases that wrack the body like arthritis or cancer. Shingles caused by the herpes virus is particularly devilish because it evades the immune system and causes pain and profound inflammation, but it is linked with another disease, chicken pox. If you never had chicken pox—and there is a childhood vaccine that prevents it—then you cannot get shingles (though you can still get chicken pox—the varicella-zoster virus, the culprit behind chicken pox and shingles, can lay dormant in your nervous system for years).

We will cover vaccines in detail in Chapter 7, but after reading about these viruses, I urge you to consider the annual vaccines available to combat them. Annual vaccines are available for other coronaviruses on the most wanted list like Middle East respiratory syndrome (MERS) and Severe Acute Respiratory Syndrome (SARS). Your annual flu shot also combats H1N1, an influenza that came out of nowhere and became an epidemic, as well as other flu viruses which mutate and change character every year to fool the immune system. These viruses are called endemic viruses—they will always be with us. Therefore, we get vaccinated yearly for infections like the flu and I suspect the same will soon be true for coronaviruses.

DR. BOB SAYS

Unless we achieve herd immunity or 70 to 80 percent exposure to a virus through vaccination or infection, we will keep feeling its effects. We don't need a global pandemic to mitigate the infections of COVID-19, its variants, and other viruses through handwashing, social distancing, and wearing a mask when required and especially when symptomatic. Get your shots and be safe so we can all live life as normally as possible! No one wants to go through what the world went through in the age of COVID-19 anytime soon.

BACTERIA WITH HIDDEN AGENDAS

Bacteria are in virtually all parts of your body—your face, genitals, underarms, bowel, lungs . . . they make up the biomes of each organ system, your skin among them. My fascination with bacteria began as a high school student, when I spent weekends growing them at a local hospital and volunteering in the bacteriology laboratory. Viruses were dead, and most hospitals cannot grow them. Bacteria seemed to have lives of their own. They had character, color in some cases, odors, and growth characteristics which assisted in their recognition and identification. They could degrade plastics, oil, and flesh. They had survived in the coldest and hottest places on earth. They colonized human organs and delivered us energy, heat, foods, drinks, and much more.

Billions of years ago, bacteria became part of each of our cells in the form of an *organelle* (little organ) called a *mitochondrion*. Life is impossible without these mitochondria, and I along with others believe that they are at the source of some of our diseases. They also inform our immune systems. Each mitochondrion is inherited solely from our mothers' eggs and are a vestigial bacterium replete with its own DNA. (Vestigial in the sense that they are vestiges of a prehistoric infection.) Our bodies have billions of these mitochondria powerhouses. They generate energy in the form of *adenosine triphosphate* (ATP), a chemical current of sorts, which is essential for every energy consuming activity that we have.

The attributes these bacteria give us while growing in our biomes, skin, lung, bowel, and kidney provide our biological soul with continuing education of a sort and are probably the greatest single source of clues to the causes of our most devastating diseases. But beyond the mitochondria and friendly invaders lurk some nasty ones. Consider Lyme disease, a common tickborne illness caused by the bacterium *Borrelia burgdorferi*. Lyme results in flu-like symptoms, rash, fatigue, and joint pain and weakness and—as with all bacteria—the chance for cross-reaction with other diseases. Lyme relies on the immune system for clearance of its spirochete, the *Borrelia*. Spirochetes are a class of bacteria that include the bad (Lyme, syphilis) and harmless (those found every day in our mouths). After all, all criminals have families; some who are criminals themselves, some completely innocent. In the case of Lyme, the body is invaded by the spirochete, which is eliminated by the immune system but not before the immune system, seeing spirochetes in certain organs like the joints, keeps ravaging the body as though the bug was in the blood.

Depending on the stage of the disease, Lyme can be eliminated from the body with adequate treatment over a few weeks, but the immune system can continue to provide symptoms, which are exceedingly difficult to treat. This difficulty has been compounded by a bit of controversy: With initial descriptions of Lyme disease, countless doctors and pharmacies spent months treating patients for the bacterium rather than realize that they were looking at what the immune system was doing to their patients. But they did it late, and the ongoing use of antibiotics for up to six months in some patients made no sense. The Lyme was gone. Huge, unnecessary antibiotic bills from medical practices with a total lack of understanding about Lyme disease is another reason why understanding the nature of what it means to be immunity strong is so important.

DR. BOB SAYS

Bacteria can be as stealthy as viruses. An infection can occur and create a whopping immune response that continues while the original bug goes on to infect someone else. A recurrent theme for bacteria and viruses is the way we misunderstand symptoms caused by our immune systems, rather than the defeated infection.

Take our next bacteria: tuberculosis (TB), an intracellular bacterial illness that likes to do what criminal viruses do: hide within the body and elude the immune system, in this case within the cells. When it wakes up, it attacks the lungs and basically eats them from the inside out, causing the chest to fill with blood. Called consumption or the white plague in the past, TB was so common that it became the subject of many great stories, including the opera *La Bohème*. But the real surprise is that it remains so common today. In fact, while there are medicines to treat it, it is still one of the world's top-ten causes of death and a permanent fixture on the antigen most wanted list.

Most of us have a TB skin test done annually to see if we have been exposed and infected, because anyone can get TB and harbor it harmlessly their entire lives. It's just that most people don't develop pulmonary TB. When they do, it is treatable, but TB is stubborn, and the medicine can take months to kill it.

Neither the medicine used to treat it nor understanding is lacking with another bacterium on the most wanted list: streptococcus. When I was studying at Rockefeller University, streptococcus was quite the subject of research by Rebecca Lancefield, a legendary scientist who identified and grouped various strains of streptococci from A to H, which today is known to all doctors around the world. The "Lancefield Criteria" of group A streptococci or strep A turned out to be one of the most important organisms with which the immune system must contend. Strep A affects millions every year, and one in five kids are strep carriers and can get strep throat repeatedly. Adults also contract strep throat—a sore throat usually accompanied by fever and swollen lymph nodes.

That strep is on the most wanted list might sound strange to many of you, especially parents reading this book who know that while highly contagious, strep throat is highly treatable with antibiotics . . . most of the time. Strep can be a master of disguise. In some people, it can cause impetigo, a certain kind of chronic kidney disease and subsequent kidney failure, and possibly (if a very sore throat is present first) *acute rheumatic fever* (RF).

RF is a condition in which your immune system reacts with your tissues because of cross reactivity with the cell wall of the strep. It produces fever, bumps under the skin, and something called migratory joint pain. It also causes extreme fatigue, jerky movements in some people, and a bizarre rash. This is rare and only happens to people whose sore throats are untreated from the outset and have the right immunogenetic predisposition. I bring it up because the cross reactivity of certain organs like the heart's valves and tissue in the brain with the wall of a miniscule bacterium like strep A is a perfect example of what we like to call *antigenic mimicry*, or confusing a bacterial antigen with a body's own tissue. It also suggests a structural similarity between some infectious agents and human proteins.

When you consider criminals, cross reactivity is analogous to master thieves changing disguises for every robbery (or even during the same robbery) so as to blend in with the surroundings and confuse their pursuers. In this case, your immune system is the pursuer. Antibodies and T cells are activated in response to the presence of the bacterial protein. Your heart valve and muscle become foreign to the immune system because of the strep's proteins, which share the same structure and are mistaken for foreign. Cytokines are released during this morass of confusion and the result is a chronic debilitating disease—not as nasty, widespread, or fatal as the nonliving insidious viruses but terrible, nonetheless.

Another bacterium that poses special problems is *Staphylococcus aureus*, better known as *staph*, which shows that bacteria like viruses do evolve, just slower than viruses. When Sir Alexander Fleming discovered penicillin in 1928—now the most widely used antibiotic in the world and responsible for saving too many lives and treating too many diseases to count—he was studying bacterial infections and (accidentally) contaminated one of his petri dishes by working next to an open window. That petri dish had staph on it from a patient and he realized that the penicillin mold prevented staph from growing. But even back then, Fleming noticed that it was effective against only one kind of staph. Today, there is a form of the staph bacteria that has adapted to the inordinate use of antibiotics and become drug-resistant: methicillin-resistant *Staphylococcus aureus* (MRSA). MRSA and other drug-resistant bacteria evolved through the (often overuse of) antibiotics and became quite common and tough to combat, wreaking havoc on patients and hospitals. MRSA infections are tough and quite common. On the one hand, new antibiotics have been developed to attack these mutants. On the other hand, no matter how sophisticated these drugs become and how much we spend to create them, bacteria will strive to fool us and eventually adapt if these drugs become overused. An ever-resistant parade of new criminal bugs will create rampant infections that the immune system is powerless to resist, which is why antibiotics cannot be the last and only stand against them in being immunity strong and why genetic approaches like CRISPR offer the most hope (see Chapter 8 for more on this).

Bacteria, particularly streptococci, have a propensity for antigenic mimicry, which confuses our immune system and makes it believe that cells and tissues might be bacterial. Certain disease manifestations can occur, which are startling and incredible—not to mention drug-resistant mutations!

But if you'll indulge my long-standing bacteria fascination, I'd like to go further down this side road of immunity strong when it comes to strep and the jerky movements I just mentioned. These movements are called *Sydenham's chorea* and are the result of re-activity of the immune system with cells within the brain—cells which have a protein that is recognized by the immune system as foreign because of similarities to the M protein of the strepto-coccus. The result is inflammation and repetitive bizarre move-ments, and one of the more interesting of these syndromes I have recorded is something I call the "Jekyll and Hyde Syndrome."

The official name of this syndrome is PANDAS, or *Pediatric Autoimmune Neuropsychiatric Disorders Associated with Streptococcal Infections*, and it is a condition in children which by observation is closest to autism than anything else that I have seen. In fact, many patients with PANDAS I have seen and studied, all affected by the syndrome between the age of three and the onset of pu-berty, have been diagnosed with "acquired autism." But PANDAS patients share one important temporal relationship besides the re-fractory and remitting symptoms mimicking autism: streptococ-cus A infection.

The first case I heard of was an eight-year-old boy who at-tempted to kill his five-year-old sister with a pair of scissors. His un-provoked and atypical behavior could not be explained by either pediatricians or pediatric psychiatrists. The only thing that had changed in his health history was he had recently endured strep throat for which he had been treated, but late. I soon saw PAN-DAS myself. The most dramatic cases were a 12-year-old girl and a 15-year-old boy who had come to see me with their respective parents. Their involuntary movements were so strange and their behavior so extreme with tics and severe obsessive-compulsive be-havior that they shocked my entire office staff. As was the case with the eight-year-old boy, the children had been normal in their behavior until they had strep.

The problem with this condition is that no amount of treatment with either glucocorticoids that inhibit the immune response or antibiotics to treat the infection have any effect on the overall behavior of the children. Many psychiatrists whom I consulted suggested that these children, while maybe not autistic, simply had OCD/tic disorders and should be considered children with psychiatric illnesses. But I don't believe that if only because *pharyngitis* (an irritation of the throat) and skin infections in a susceptible child causes an abnormal immune response with central nervous system manifestations. Everyone seems to agree on that, and it does relate back to Sydenham's chorea. The fundamental question is whether the immune system is responding to the chronic strep infection by making antibodies and causing this abnormal behavior.

While the role of autoimmunity in these children is extremely controversial, it could give some credence to the immune basis of behavioral problems in children and the idea being explored in scientific journals that we touched on in Chapter 2 and that autism is an autoimmune disorder. Imagine if this streptococcal cross-reactive abnormal behavior leads us to the true cause of this untreatable and perhaps misunderstood malady. Imagine if behavior problems in children were linked to strong immune responses!

WHAT ABOUT PARASITES?

One summer in college, I was privileged to work as an animal attendant at a large pharmaceutical company that was developing antiparasitic drugs for sheep. Certain parasites are devastating to animals in countries like Australia, which depend on the sheep industry. Veterinary surgeons developed a novel way to see if worms were eliminated: They sewed faucets with valves to the stomachs of sheep, which I was required to empty daily. It was an easy way to see the burden of infection, how well drugs worked, how well the immune system of the sheep worked, and it was also quite an introduction to these criminals.

Parasites are organisms that live on or in us and feed on our cells and tissues to survive. There are many parasitic diseases wreaking havoc in the world and all of them are doing so through the immune system. One of the most common is malaria, a disease caused by a plasmodium parasite transmitted by the bite of an infected mosquito. Malaria begins with flu-like symptoms, and when untreated leads to progressive disease causing hundreds of thousands of deaths every year. The vast majority of malaria cases come from sub-Saharan Africa and South Asia, and while sickle cells developed in Africans as a Darwinian adaptation to prevent death from malaria, others have no resistance. Travelers to these areas often take antiparasitic chemical agents or antimalarial drugs to prevent it.

Other most wanted parasitic criminals have no drugs to prevent them. The deadliest have horrible names and do even more horrible things, like *naegleria fowleri*, the brain-eating amoeba. Many of these parasites are exceedingly rare and are largely found outside the United States in tropical and developing countries. But not all. Tickborne diseases like *ehrlichiosis* and *babesiosis* are common in this hemisphere as is *Chagas disease*, which is transmitted through the bite of a triatomine fly and infects hundreds of thousands of people in the Americas every year. It can cause digestive and neurological problems and especially cardiac complications. Most people who die from the infection suffer heart attacks.

DR. BOB SAYS

Parasites that cause infection, like worms, malaria, and amoebae used to be rare but since air travel can bring us anywhere in the world in a day, they are less rare than before. Like all antigen criminals, these invaders can be stealthy and live with us without knowledge.

The good news is Chagas disease and most parasitic diseases are treatable with antiparasitic drugs. The bad news is, like all invaders, they are often difficult to diagnose and treat, so we use our knowledge of the immune system to find them and kill them. This is possible because parasitic infections use a whole different array of cells, cytokines, and antibodies than other infections. It's as though a criminal parasitic infection calls out to the immune system's version of special police that most of us don't know exists on a day-to-day basis like Amtrak or United States Postal Service officers. For example, if a parasitic worm is acquired from eating infected meat, a group of cells known as mast cells—basophilic cells, and most importantly eosinophilic (typically a form of white cell) cells—accumulate and attack the parasite along with a special antibody called IgE. The whole attack is very efficient, but like those real-life officers, these are not police that are prepared for an infection of scale and are often overwhelmed with the degree of infection.

Once again, modern medicine has stepped up to support the immune system with those drugs that work against most parasites. But there will always be more. The antigen most wanted list will never be exhausted. If you have learned anything in this chapter, I hope it is that infections have mastered the nuances of immunity and know how to take advantage of your immune system in the most sophisticated ways. If an infection can bypass normal processes by entering a cell and hiding, disrupting, or killing a specific cell type, or announcing itself with fanfare after colossal entry into cells and organs, your immune system can fail. Antibiotics, antiviral agents, vaccines, and other therapies have helped stem the tide but not always. Of course, not all infections are acute, and organisms have learned to adapt to help us, and in some cases protect us by informing our immune system. But we must be vigilant and keep understanding more about what lives within us and what they do to us.

Remember: If your biological soul gives in, you die.

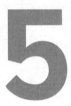

5 Autoimmunity and Anarchy

Jillian was 23 when she arrived at my clinic: red, blistered, nauseous, sleepless for two days, and miserable from the sunburn she had gotten after two weeks at the beach with her friends. None of those conditions were unusual for a sunburn as severe as hers. What was unusual was the severe joint pain throughout her body and her malaise (general feeling of discomfort and inability to function). She did not think this had anything to do with her "sun poisoning." Neither did I. Several tests and a clinical exam confirmed what I suspected: Jillian had the same disease as Corliss, whose story opened Chapter 1: *systemic lupus erythematosus*, or lupus, an autoimmune disease that can be triggered, for reasons unknown, by excessive sun exposure.

I used to believe that the worst thing that one could get from too much sun was skin cancer. Not for people like Jillian. Treating her lupus was a matter of life and death. Her immune system was attacking her body, a process called *autoimmunity*.

To be clear, autoimmunity is part of our normal biology. We all go about our day with some normal autoimmune responses that result in the development of autoantibodies (blood proteins that react with one's own tissues) and produce nothing that we recognize as abnormal. Occasionally, self-reactive lymphocytes mature and can be activated to cause autoimmune disease, but generally your innate immunity successfully screens its new cell "recruits" to differentiate self from nonself. As we touched on at the start of this book, the problem is when your immune system's first responders suddenly believe your body is the criminal—from a resourceful virus like COVID-19 or an autoimmune disease like lupus. Your innate immunity fails to do what it has been able to do since you were born—recognize self from nonself or correctly identify the good guys from the bad guys. Some call this autoimmunity a form of immunodeficiency because the immune system's T cells and B cells do not function in the appropriate manner. Others refer to it as a hyperimmune state because the immune system seems to be attacking everything and considers organs and tissues foreign antigens, sometimes without regard for the damage that results.[1]

I have made the study of autoimmune disease a major part of my life, and I call it one word: anarchy. Yes, anarchy.

Anarchy is defined as the absence of order. But in autoimmunity your body's state of disorder is not due to absence of authority; it's an assault by the first responders sworn to protect you from invaders like viruses, bacteria, and parasites. In autoimmunity those first responders have turned against you. *Anything and everything* can be a criminal in these autoimmune situations and your first responders—sensing danger from within—attack your organs and tissues.

I presented one example of this anarchy in Chapter 1 when Greg contracted COVID-19 and ended up fighting for his life through a cytokine storm. Like Greg, Jillian had been perfectly healthy

---

[1] Curiously, diseases in the immune system seem to prefer certain organs in certain people for no obvious reason. One patient can have a skin disease and another kidney disease. It was such an issue that I thought at one point that lupus was many diseases under one name.

before her sun exposure triggered her autoimmune response. Her condition was stable but dire. She was in great pain and could go into heart or kidney failure depending on the severity of her autoimmune condition and the organs her disease chose. Would it lead to anarchy? That's the first question this chapter answers. The rest of this chapter digs deeper into autoimmune anarchy, including possible connections to brain disorders and even cancer, so not only how the whole process of the determination of self might be imperfect but that maybe, autoimmunity has a purpose. All this knowledge is essential to being immunity strong and understanding the mysteries of the biological soul.

DR. BOB SAYS

Autoimmunity happens in our bodies as a normal process. It is not a harmful thing until a disease develops. But it is possible that autoimmunity is a major aspect of inflammation and consequently at the heart of our most common diseases like those affecting the heart, lungs, and brain.

THE MYSTERIES OF AUTOIMMUNITY

When Jillian presented in our clinic, we did a thorough examination and tested her blood and urine. The examination revealed that she had a "rub" in her chest—a noise that sounds like two pieces of leather being rubbed together. The tests revealed a frothy pink urine. Both were alarming. The rub could have been the apposition of two layers of tissue; in this case, the coverings of her heart. The same complexes causing problems with the heart lining could also be in her joints and wreaking havoc with pain and inflammation. The frothy pink urine could mean that she already had complexes of antibodies deposited on her kidney membranes, punching holes in them, and causing blood and protein to "leak" into her urine. All these symptoms did not indicate an all-out assault, but it was anarchical as Jillian's immune system attacked cells and tissues that it should not. Jillian could go into heart or kidney failure based on these findings and their severity.

In this situation, you might think of Jillian's first responders as people vandalizing and looting stores in their own neighborhoods. It doesn't seem to make any sense and any explanations are incomplete at best. The plan of treatment is the same, however: Turn down the volume as quickly as possible without fanning the proverbial flames. For Jillian, that required an understanding of how lupus and autoimmune diseases work.

The first known documented case of lupus dates back to the father of modern medicine, Hippocrates. The word *lupus* (which means "wolf" in Latin) dates back to the thirteenth century. But the history of the study of autoimmunity is much more recent. It starts with Paul Ehrlich, a 1909 Nobel Prize–winning scientist whose research helped establish the field of immunology. Ehrlich coined the term *horror autotoxicus*, or the horror of self-toxicity, and most of his findings were descriptive, since immunity as a science was fairly rudimentary during his lifetime. While he correctly described our innate immunity's ability to sort self from nonself, he resisted the concept of autoimmunity and the immune system ever attacking itself. Ehrlich was so influential that it wasn't until 1957 that the idea that (newly discovered) autoantibodies and the immune system attacking itself were considered as causes of many autoimmune diseases we now treat.

The spectrum of autoimmunity is huge and is divided into autoimmune diseases that are systemic (anything in the body might be a target) or organ-specific (involving only one or possibly two organs). Familiar autoimmune diseases that target organs or systems include type I diabetes (insulin dependence from birth), multiple sclerosis (where the insulation of nerves is destroyed), Graves' disease (which impacts the thyroid), vitiligo (loss of pigment in the skin), and myasthenia gravis (antibodies to the muscle receptors that make them work), and the chronic systemic autoimmune diseases like rheumatoid arthritis, scleroderma, and Jillian's systemic lupus erythematosus, which defy cause and affect multiple organs.[2]

Lupus affects about five million people (mostly women) worldwide and the symptoms can be far less severe than Jillian's and mitigated by treatment. So, why give it such prominence? Because lupus is the prototypical autoimmune disease. It has features of many other autoimmune diseases—rheumatoid arthritis, multiple sclerosis, scleroderma, Sjogren's syndrome, diabetes, and encephalitis. We call lupus a multisystemic disease because it affects almost any organ of the body; the organs that are likely to be affected are the kidneys, brain, and skin (and more rarely the heart and lungs). The antibodies found in this disease are as numerous as food on a giant buffet. The immune and other responses are also incredibly varied: there are many antibodies as T cell and B cell abnormalities—all targets for therapy in Jillian and for research and drug development for society.

As we cover in the next chapter, pharmaceutical companies have huge budgets to understand the process of autoimmunity and develop medications like anti-cytokine drugs or engineered monoclonal antibodies known as biologicals, which will regulate your immune system and prevent any anarchy from destroying your organs. Some of these drugs—and not just those designed

---

[2] There are some bizarre autoimmune conditions that have piqued my interest over the years. For instance, some natural medicines like hormones can cause autoimmunity. One peculiar condition is a skin condition called dermatitis, which occurs in women who have lots of the hormone progesterone in their blood. It is caused by the injection of 19 alpha hydroxyprogesterone to treat preterm labor in pregnant women. Another unusual condition involves autoimmunity to bodily fluids like semen, which can occur in some women as well as men. The basic proteins in semen can become antigenic and in bad cases precipitate anaphylactic shock. This is reported to have happened in several instances where a woman after intercourse was found to have hives and shortness of breath. In men it is most noticeable after ejaculation when there may be severe itching or burning along the shaft of the penis. Sometimes nausea, fever, and bodily rash can be components of this condition, which should be treated as soon as possible. (It is possible to be desensitized to the semen for both men and women, but it is a long and tedious process.)

to treat autoimmune diseases—can even trigger autoimmunity if given to a patient with the wrong illness. For example, I've found that drug-induced autoimmunity in someone getting a cytokine inhibitor for rheumatoid arthritis can actually induce a lupus-like illness.

Regular nonbiological medications can do the same thing. One of my first papers for the *New England Journal of Medicine* was about Hans, a 63-year-old school principal. Hans had been hospitalized for an irregular heartbeat. The cardiologists managed his care and placed him on procainamide to regularize his heart rate. Procainamide is usually a wonderful drug that can regularize the heart rhythm, but after two weeks, Hans developed profound joint pain, a fiery red rash over his face, and a feeling that someone had beat his body to a pulp. He was admitted to the hospital, but the doctors did not connect what perhaps you did because of Jillian's story: that he had an autoimmune condition, specifically drug-induced lupus or autoimmunity. All because Hans was an older man and did not fit the profile. Testing, however, suggested an autoimmune condition that looked like "drug-induced lupus," a condition triggered by certain drugs that either become foreign to the body themselves or provoke some sort of chemical response that remains unknown. In Hans, procainamide, an activated amine, caused the disease, and when it was removed from his system, the volume was turned down, order was restored, and he completely recovered.

For Jillian, whose lupus diagnosis was more obvious, a different approach was taken to turn down the volume and restore some order in the anarchy inside her. First, since she clearly had renal failure, we quickly did a kidney biopsy to see how much damage immune complexes had done and a skin biopsy to see why her rash was so bright red and painful. After reviewing the results, we determined she needed to be put on *hydroxychloroquine* (an immunosuppressive drug) and *prednisone* (corticosteroids for her rash). She did not need the cytotoxic drugs (usually drugs used in chemotherapy) reserved for extremely sick patients because their side effects are often untenable. With significant immunosuppression, Jillian did quite well and was discharged with a recommendation of bed rest and plenty of fluids to protect her organs. Within two weeks, she felt normal again.

But the treatment of Jillian (and Hans) only covers *what* happens when treating patients for autoimmune diseases like lupus. The *why* still eludes us. Even after 50 years of research on lupus, we still don't understand why sunlight causes patients like Jillian to develop and flare with the disease or why lupus disproportionately affects women of childbearing age. Understanding autoimmunity allows us to suspect which organs are being subverted by the immune system but still leaves us with the fundamental question dealing with autoimmunity: *Why does it attack and select certain organs—why the kidneys in Jillian or the brain in someone else?*

The answers are as varied as they are elusive. A popular thought for drug-induced autoimmunity (one that I and many others subscribe to) is that it is an epigenetic condition or temporary heritable change in gene expression. In Hans's case, this was brought about by a medicine that regularized the patient's heartbeat but caused an autoimmune disease at the same time by producing metabolites that changed the expression of his genes. The questions surrounding epigenetic drug and toxin effects on the human body and the subsequent appearance of autoimmune disease are both intriguing and vexing simply because the mechanisms are not known.

Most scientists and physicians believe that there is an inheritance to autoimmunity, but it is not obvious and not inherited via Mendel's genetic principles. (Mendel, genetics, and epigenetics are covered in depth in Chapter 8.) They are also not inherited like Huntington's disease or sickle cell anemia, though they are associated with transplantation genes or the MHC (major histocompatibility complex) on chromosome 6, which rules your immune system. Lupus also offers some additional clues. The fact that lupus only occurs in 50 percent or less of identical twins could mean that there are environmental factors that are important. Meanwhile, mice who are affected by systemic lupus often have genetic defects that predispose them to the illness.

There are lots of other genetic defects leading to autoimmunity, too: defective clearance of an antigen from the blood from dead cells; a failure of programmed cell death brought on by a toxin, a hormone, or organism; or the abundance of cytokines or chemical messengers to various cells in the body during and after an infection. Infections can be particularly devious criminals as they recruit and activate innocent bystanders (lymphocytes) as accomplices to act autoreactive when the infectious organisms are in the body. Consider rheumatic fever and Lyme disease, in which the infection activates an autoimmune response, sometimes vigorous and sometimes mild. When doctors treat rheumatic fever and Lyme, we realize that we are no longer dealing with the organisms that caused the problem. When a lingering condition occurs after the bugs are gone or dead, we are dealing with autoimmunity (probably a lasting immune response). There is also a condition called iatrogenic autoimmunity or immunity caused by us, your doctors. For instance, anticancer drugs like flucloxacillin can cause antibodies to appear, which react with tumors. Drugs like these cause a loss of what we call tolerance and induce an antibody response against you and me.

Finally, induced autoimmunity is not limited to chemical drugs. A young doctor died after receiving a COVID-19 vaccine in the early days of the roll out. He bled to death after the vaccine caused the loss of platelets (a major component in normal blood clotting). In fact, his platelets were zero when he died. The reason for the death of this doctor and several other cases of autoimmune-induced attacks on platelets unrelated to vaccinations are probably the unmasking of a genetic error or defect that leads to *thrombocytopenia* (low platelets), which is difficult to overcome but can be treated. This applied to the pause in the administration AstraZeneca and Johnson & Johnson COVID-19 vaccines in 2021 when there were very rare cases of venous clots in the brain and a total loss of platelets with extreme hemorrhage (though only a few of those affected died).

In conclusion, I am convinced that autoimmunity is at the basis of many diseases that drive us mad in medicine. Everything from accelerated atherosclerosis to dementia may be autoimmune in part, some say due to inflammation, or the remnants of past infections. One of the most important and interesting aspects of autoimmunity is when it affects the most immunologically privileged organ in your body: your brain.

DR. BOB SAYS

Many of our most common diseases are autoimmune or involve autoimmune features. Multiple sclerosis, type 1 diabetes, lupus, rheumatoid arthritis, and many others involve your immune system and its reaction with "self." We can't prevent these rogue antibodies and cells, but we can control them.

THE BRAIN AND AUTOIMMUNITY

Jillian had a systemic autoimmune disease rather than single-organ-specific autoimmunity. Organ-specific rheumatic diseases are peculiar, because the reason for the autoimmune attack on specific organs are not clear. This is even less clear and much more problematic than lupus when the attack is on the brain. When the immune system attacks the brain, the changes are often permanent.

Immunological privilege refers to areas within the body that escape recognition by the body as self for many years. We first encountered the brain as a privileged site in Chapter 2 on biomes. I called it a gated community with its own first responders. The gate is actually a blood-brain barrier that keeps the cellular riffraff out. But while the brain is the most prominent gated community in your body, it is not the only one. The eye, testicle, thyroid, and uterus/fetus are other privileged sites with limited access to the peripheral immune system. Cytokines and chemokines can act in these privileged areas without difficulty, but when your natural killer T cells venture into them, there is no destruction, and tolerance is quickly induced. In fact, many antigens that are expressed in these privileged sites induce neither tolerance nor activation of the immune system. But some are often targeted by it. For example, in multiple sclerosis *myelin basic protein*, the insulation around the nerves in the brain, becomes antigenic. Or look at *Hashimoto thyroid disease* (inflammation of the thyroid or thyroiditis). Named for Dr. Hakaru Hashimoto, a Japanese physician and medical scientist of the Meiji and Taisho periods in Japan, antibodies in this condition attack the thyroid, causing it to become enlarged, slow down, or even cease to function and leading to fatigue and weight gain in young women.

That said, when the activation of the immune system happens outside the privileged areas, they can become targets for autoimmune attack. For example, if your eyeball is injured as a result of some trauma (say, getting hit hard by a ball), sequestered privileged antigens are released as a result of the inflammation and confront lymph nodes and T cells. When immune responses mounted against the antigen from the injured eye meet the protected antigen of the other non-injured eye, an immune attack of the non-injured eye happens, called *sympathetic ophthalmia*.

Fascinating stuff. Interest in these topics, especially the brain-peripheral immune system connection, has given rise to neuro-immunology, a remarkable specialty that studies mental diseases like schizophrenia, bipolar disorder, and depression because of an immune insult to the brain. Dr. Tsuyoshi Miyaoka, a Japanese psychiatrist, tells a story that is perfectly illustrative of this specialty. A 23-year-old man came to Miyaoka, convinced his thoughts were leaking out of his head, that other people were listening to him, and that his radiator spoke to him. He was anxious, could not sleep, and felt at times he could not go on with life. The patient was diagnosed and treated as a paranoid schizophrenic and prescribed a series of antipsychotic drugs. Nothing helped. The year after the patient's diagnosis, he developed a cancer of the blood called *acute myeloid leukemia*. To survive, he needed a bone marrow transplant. After the procedure, his delusions and paranoia completely disappeared. His schizophrenia had vanished.

We know bone marrow transplants during cancer treatment essentially revitalize the immune system. Chemotherapy kills off your old white blood cells, and all sorts of new cells sprout from the stem cells in the donor's transplanted bone marrow. In the case of this man's immune system, it was apparently driving his psychiatric condition, and when it was revitalized, so was he. According to Moises Velasquez-Manoff, author of *An Epidemic of Absence: A New Way to Understand Allergies and Autoimmune Diseases*, this theory that the immune system is the root of many mental illnesses has a long history. For example, in the late nineteenth-century, physicians noticed that when infections tore through psychiatric wards, the resulting fevers (called *hyperpyrexia*) caused an improvement in the conditions of mentally ill and even catatonic patients. After the fever subsided, the disorders returned. Similarly, Dr. Julius Wagner-Jauregg, an Austrian physician winner of the 1927 Nobel Prize, developed a method of delivering the malaria parasite to psychiatric patients to induce a fever. While many patients died of the infection, many recovered completely without psychiatric complaints.

On the flip side, there are numerous examples of patients having psychotic disease associated with autoimmunity, including Susannah Cahalan, a friend and editor at the *New York Post* who wrote a book about her diagnosis called *Brain on Fire*. Susannah had experienced a very rare psychiatric condition called *NMDA receptor autoimmune encephalitis*. (The antigen NMDA is a channel protein in nerve cells known to be a cause of psychosis in patients who make antibodies against it. In the brain, it is an enzyme that is fundamental to behavior.) Susannah became totally psychotic with terrifying symptoms like paranoia, homicidal thoughts, and an inability to do any executive activities. Lucky for her, a neurologist diagnosed her correctly in spite of the fact she was only the 217th person in the world to be documented with this disorder.

She received a concoction of corticosteroids, immunoglobulin infusions, and plasmapheresis (blood exchange), which she credits for her recovery. I shudder to think of the patients who fail to get this diagnosis and have been incarcerated in mental institutions.

Personally, I have observed patients with autoimmune diseases who have problems with behavior, transient psychosis, and altered personality like the lupus Jillian had or Sjogren's syndrome (an autoimmune disease I call the "desert syndrome" because it attacks the tear glands of the eyes, mucous membranes, and glands that make saliva and produces dry eyes and mouth). These are conditions replete with antibodies, shifts in cells, and the synthesis of many cytokines and chemokines. I have always thought that this was autoimmunity attacking the patient's brain and, in a condition called *neuropsychiatric lupus*, and this turned out to be the case. (Curiously, we found no anatomical or histological changes within those brains through imaging or autopsy.) Beyond my own work, experts in the field of neuroimmunology have linked immunity to depression, bipolar disorder, and even eating disorders. There has also been the discovery of specific antibodies against cells within the nervous system that would cause *dystonia* or bizarre muscle tone within the body.

One of the more interesting conditions that may be associated with the immune system and brain antigens is autism. There are no specific antigens like neurofilaments, myelin basic protein, or other neuronal cells that have been targeted by antibodies in autistic children and most of the findings are not specific to autism. Many investigators consider a lack of oxygen or an immunological insult within the uterus of the pregnant mother as a possible causative factor of autism, but no one seems to be sure. Which is why, as an immunologist, I tend to look where others do not: the peripheral immune system.

In Chapter 2, I noted that some children with autism have some strange biomes and unusual organisms in their stool and discussed PANDAS or pediatric autoimmune neuropsychiatric disorder associated with streptococcal infections as an example of an infection and immune response that creates a condition analogous to autism in young children. (OCD, flailing extremities, and outright bizarre behavior soon after a strep infection.) Sydenham's chorea and PANDAS are also autoimmune attacks on neurons that cause strange movements and behavior with normal mentation. Here, when it comes to autoimmunity, I will note that some autistic children also have increased incidence of autoimmune diseases and their relatives, immunoglobulin deficiencies, and increased autoantibodies. The research is waiting to be done by investigators who accept the challenge.

Autism is an admittedly charged developmental condition, but no matter what you believe, I will intentionally repeat myself here and again in the vaccine chapter: Vaccinations are *not* linked to autism even though this continues to be the *cause célèbre* of "anti-vaxxers." But while the autism-vaccine link is worthless, I am encouraged by possible links to autoimmunity—and not just autism. A link between autoimmunity and cancer might be of incredible value to our future understanding of this behavioral exception.

DR. BOB SAYS

Autoimmunity has been involved as a cause of mental diseases like schizophrenia and depression. There is also evidence that conditions like dementia and autism might have autoimmune mechanisms in their origins.

AUTOIMMUNITY AND CANCER

A young woman named Ling knew something was terribly wrong with her. She could barely open her mouth. She had problems swallowing. Her hands almost always felt cold and numb. Her stool was loose. When Ling's doctor, a rheumatologist, added exceptionally high blood pressure to her list of symptoms, his suspicions were that Ling had a condition called progressive systemic sclerosis or *scleroderma* (an autoimmune rheumatic disease that attacks the skin and connective tissues). Scleroderma can be associated with high blood pressure, extreme weight loss due to thickened bowel and malabsorption, difficulty swallowing, Raynaud's syndrome (a painful constriction of blood vessels in the hands and the feet that leads to an extreme color response to cold and severe stress), and curious darkening of the skin. Ling had all of these things. Confident of his clinical diagnosis, the doctor opted to test Ling for specific antibodies that would confirm his diagnosis without putting her through a biopsy. When she tested positive for antibodies to *RNA polymerase III*, he had no doubt. Patients who have antibodies to RNA polymerase III have a particularly aggressive form of scleroderma.

Ling's scleroderma diagnosis was par for the course for a good rheumatologist, even for a fairly rare disease. What was interesting was the possible connection to the cancerous tumor that also turned up. Ling had a kidney tumor that was secreting cytokines and there were other growth factors that resulted in her thickened skin. A scan of Ling's abdomen revealed the renal mass, and she had a nephrectomy (removal of her one diseased kidney). Ling survived the cancer, and my colleagues at Johns Hopkins University published a paper in *Science* in which they hypothesized that scleroderma and perhaps other autoimmune diseases might be part of the body's ferocious battle to fend off cancer—that the anarchy of autoimmunity is a casualty of war between cancer and the immune system. Their hypothesis went like this: Cancer mutates a normal gene that produces a protein that causes an immune response, and that immune response leads to the disease scleroderma. The hypothesis was based on the fact that autoimmune diseases like *myositis* (inflammation of muscle) or Sjogren's syndrome predispose patients to cancers. That led them to the idea that maybe the immune response was targeting a form of the molecule present in the patient's tumor.

Could this response be part of the why that has eluded us when it comes to the purpose of autoimmunity? Might this lead to an immunologic cure for cancer?

Tumors are insidious groups of renegade cells—terrorists, really—that hijack organs and eventually grow large enough to become resistant to the normal immune response. I will never forget a professor in medical school saying we develop tumors within our bodies all the time, but they are small-time crooks—microscopic collections of cells which our innate first responders easily clear. So, cancers continuously try to evolve into better criminals and avoid detection by whatever the immune system's first responders are throwing at it. This hypothesis regarding immune surveillance and cancer trying to avoid detection is credited to Dr. Antony Rosen, director of rheumatology and vice dean for research at Johns Hopkins Medical School. Dr. Rosen theorized that over time, cancer does something that the immune system cannot attack. This is especially true as we get older. Elderly people lose this immune surveillance in the inevitable aging of immunity or immunosenescence, when their immune response gets suppressed, but the cancer keeps moving forward and eventually kills the patient unchecked. Emotional responses to catastrophic events might also depress immune surveillance. For example, there are many stories about cancers developing after the death of a loved one.

When a tumor does escape detection and starts to grow, it closes itself off like a cult guarding its compound inside your body. Your first responders have failed to detect or deal with the tumor, so they need outside help once it is detected. Chemotherapy and radiation are the most common approaches, though they can be debilitating and some cancers like prostate and pancreatic do not respond to it. There are monoclonal antibodies that can attack tumors from breast, lung, or colon cancer. We also have drugs like Rituxan that lower the numbers of B cells in lymphomas caused by them. Immunotherapy has elicited durable clinical responses and in a fraction of patients produced long-term remission of tumors, with no signs of cancer for many years. The novel nature of these new drugs is that they involve an antibody against two markers blocking a T cell response. They do not target the tumor cell, but they target the molecules involved in the protection of the tumor cell.

But in spite of all these advances, cancer remains a crafty most wanted criminal. That's because regulation of T cell responses is extremely complex, consisting of both stimulation and inhibition of pathways that limit the T cell responses against the cancer. Once T cells go near and enter a tumor, they face all kinds of restrictions: T cells that act against them, suppressor cells that come from the bone marrow and appear without warning, cytokines that inhibit the actions of T cells, and other cells in the complex tumor network. All these restrictions act against the immune system's attack on the tumor. The tumor also elicits its own protective antigens that keeps the T cells away.

Why the immune system does this and in all its brilliance fails to combat cancer remains a question every immunologist has asked themselves at some point. As we will learn in the next chapter, two Nobel Prize–winning scientists did more than ask this question; they found a way to answer it using monoclonal antibodies or biologicals, which fight fire with fire.

Can autoimmunity play a role in the cause and cure of cancer? Science is exploring that! Fundamental questions revolve around the fact that antibodies are made against parts of cells for no reason like DNA, RNA, and organelles. These antibodies to "self" are intriguing and might offer us clues to figure out many of the mysteries that affect medicine today.

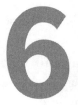

6 Inflammation, Biologicals, and Fighting Fire with Fire

Like many moms, Samantha got up before her children and made them breakfast before school. Unlike those moms, Samantha woke up extra early to take five or six anti-inflammatory medications in large doses—at first aspirin, then ibuprofen—in order to do that much. Until her late 30s, Sam had been the ultimate soccer mom. Now 40, she dreamed of just taking her four kids to school without being in constant pain. Every morning, she woke up fatigued and remained stiff for hours. Depending on the weather, she might not be able to walk. What made things worse was that Sam had no clue as to the cause of her illness until her doctor suspected rheumatoid arthritis (RA), a chronic inflammatory disorder, and referred her to a rheumatologist.

The year was 2011. If Sam had been treated by most rheumatologists for RA a few decades earlier, she would have been put on narcotics to manage the pain, given injections of cortisone (a synthetic corticosteroid or steroid hormone mentioned in the last chapter), and/or large doses of nonsteroidal anti-inflammatory drugs (NSAIDs). She might also get injections of gold and be advised to wear a copper bracelet. Those treatments would have left Sam with deformity, bone erosion, and disability, specifically an inability to walk or use her hands, by the time she turned 50. But in 2011, Sam's rheumatologist was able to get her onto a class of drugs called biologicals—drugs that employ natural substances like antibodies to control infections and inflammation to treat rheumatoid arthritis and other immune diseases and prevent the destruction of organs like the heart and lungs. Using these engineered biological mini missiles known as *monoclonal antibodies*, he said, "We are fighting fire with fire. You are going to feel so good you'll be able to run a 10K race."

The effectiveness of these remarkable guided missiles to help our biological soul has come of age, providing molecular therapies that are revolutionizing medicine. Pharmaceutical companies have billion-dollar budgets for developing biologicals like engineered monoclonal antibodies (proteins designed to target specific antigens or even parts of an antigenic molecule) and anti-cytokine drugs (which target the communication molecules of the immune system) to combat a variety of immune, autoimmune, and inflammatory diseases. The more common the disease, the greater the push to treat them, which is why many medications in the field of rheumatology are directed toward RA. It is not only debilitating, but also the most common autoimmune disease in the world, affecting about 1 percent of the worldwide population—nearly eight million people—and taxing the economies of individuals, families, and even nations.

If you have ever seen an advertisement for one of these medications, sometimes there are trade-offs to these advances; the side effects listed are often numerous and would be comical if they weren't so awful. Some even risk disturbing the body's homeostatic mechanisms. Nonetheless, the appearance of biologicals has been nothing short of revolutionary, earning Nobel Prizes and making clinicians like me incredibly grateful.

This chapter explores the evolution of this "hot" topic among immunologists today: fighting fire with fire—the movement away from chemical-based drugs to biologicals and using the immune system to control itself and keep you healthy. We will understand how monoclonal antibodies came to be and the revolutionary strides they have made in attacking diseases like RA and even cancer. But first, we must take a deeper dive into the fire those biologicals often fight—inflammation.

INFLAMMATION AND THE IMMUNE SYSTEM

Everyone experiences inflammation at some point in their lives: infections, bruises, cuts, splinters ... all these perpetrators produce the pain, redness, limited immobility, flushed feeling, low-grade fever, swelling, and tenderness commonly associated with acute inflammation. These feelings are short-term, unpleasant, and usually minor.

As we learned at the start of this book, those acute inflammatory reactions are the work of your innate immune response sounding an alarm and catching the bad guys at the crime scene before they can do any real harm. What is literally going on when you experience acute inflammation involves the movement of blood plasma and groups of cells called *phagocytes* (monocytes and, more specifically, macrophages, granulocytes, and dendritic cells). The phagocytes hear the call from your cytokine and chemokine communication network and work together help your immune system fight off infection.

The name *phagocyte* comes from the Greek word for "eat," and that is exactly what these cells do: They eat and cart away any bad guys that caused the inflammation in your body. It starts with the cells already residing in your tissues: macrophages, dendritic cells, others like histiocytes and mast cells working to employ those pattern recognition receptor proteins (alarmins and defensins). The main purpose of these cells is to recognize damage or an invasion of your tissue by criminal external pathogens—viruses, bacteria, parasites—or objects like splinters, nails, or perhaps a burn from a pot on the stove (and not "arrest" normal cells, which might lead to bigger problems).

When an invasion is detected, these cells activate and release chemicals that are responsible for the inflammatory reaction: The blood vessels dilate and increased blood flow occurs, which causes redness and increased fluid accumulation. The porosity of the blood vessels allows the macrophage and granulocyte phagocytes to go into the tissue. The blood vessels then begin to leak plasma proteins and fluid, which goes into the tissue, causing the swelling you experience. Some of these inflammatory mediators, such as *bradykinin* or *histamine*, result in the increased sensitivity and nerve pain you might have at the site of the inflammation.

As a rule, these phagocytes are only in the blood vessel circulation and not allowed to enter the tissues of the body. But this is a special event. Signals have gone out from the area of injury, like an all-points bulletin to your first responders from those cytokines and chemokines. That's when the inflammation at the scene of the crime starts looking like a biological motor vehicle accident. Other chemicals have been activated in attempts to heal you like the *complement system* (which amplifies your immune response by enhancing the ability of phagocytic cells to do their work) and the *coagulation cascade* (which allows the removal of blood and the clotting off of small vessels to prevent spread of whatever caused the inflammation). If all goes well, your neutrophils—those white blood cells that eat germs and carry them away like the paddy wagons—carry the captured criminals away from the scene, and the inflammation, possibly with the help of a local antiseptic, disappears anywhere from a few hours to a few days later.

DR. BOB SAYS

That skin infection that spreads up and around your leg or arm, resulting in fever and pain? That's a kind of inflammation, and inflammation is our friend! Redness, pain, fever, and swelling are all part of an organized chaos that is a normal reaction of your immune system designed to protect you. It is natural and reflects your body's attempt to control what would otherwise cause true damage to your health or even kill you.

Of course, some acute inflammation requires more than a topical ointment or simple course of pain medications and antibiotics. For example, while many viruses only produce a short-term fever, when the antigen virus is COVID-19 and the acute inflammation occurs within a specific organ (most commonly the lung, as it was with Greg in Chapter 1), we strive at the outset of the infection to provide the patient with large doses of corticosteroids like dexamethasone and flood the system with a large amount of anti-inflammatory hormone, which may make the difference between life and death. Or consider HIV and the CD4 T cell depletion and disease caused by the virus. Those inflammatory events propel patients toward AIDS, where there is initial inflammation and then "silence" since the immune system is dysfunctional. Research efforts to create a lifetime course of medications to control that inflammation are at the heart of controlling the immune response to save the patient.[1]

That said, you know from Sam's story that acute inflammation is not the only kind of inflammation. Prolonged or chronic inflammation, long-term inflammation produced by infection, injury, or diseases like RA, lead to a progressive shift in phagocytic cells present at the site of inflammation, and monocytes such as the macrophages and the dendritic cells. The resulting inflammation is characterized by a simultaneous destruction and healing of tissue from the inflammatory process, and a kind of remodeling and repair that happens over and over again. Think of it as your first responders reacting to a burglar alarm going off again and again. Every time it happens, your immune system produces those cells and chemicals and, in some cases, even attacks itself, which is what we learned happens in autoimmune diseases.

No matter what kind of inflammation you have, it is important to understand two things moving forward. First, inflammation is

---

[1] Curiously, in AIDS patients, there is a condition called "reconstitution syndrome," which is where there is illness and inflammation when the immune system is rejuvenated with treatment. The newer HIV medicines can cause this syndrome.

not synonymous with infection because inflammation can occur without infection. Inflammation is your body's immunovascular response to any cause, be it a broken bone or antigen. Second, inflammation is not synonymous with pain. In my practice, I see patients with back and foot pain; repetitive stress injuries to their wrists or fingers; or varieties of pain syndromes involving their muscles or joints. Their pain is unassociated with inflammation. This is part of the reason why every patient we see is tested for an elevation of *acute phase reactants* (the erythrocyte sedimentation rate and the C-reactive protein). When these do not exist in the presence of severe pain throughout the body, that's a problem, because it indicates that classical inflammation is not present. It is only when fatigue, a neighbor to pain, is present that the immunologist in me gets concerned, as fatigue is often a determinant of inflammation somewhere in the body. And when it comes to autoimmune diseases like RA, inflammation and pain are horribly, debilitatingly linked, which is why the first drugs to fight that fire were so important.

DR. BOB SAYS

Having pain is not synonymous with inflammation. Substances make inflammation happen in response to a stimulus. This inflammation is generally associated with cells moving in and out of a specific area of the body. It can happen in your joints, under the skin, and in organs like the heart, lungs, and brain.

THE FIRST FIGHTS AGAINST FIRE

For many decades, folks like Sam with RA had only one course of treatment for their chronic inflammation: steroids—specifically a steroid hormone called cortisone, a kind of *corticosteroid* (or *glucocorticoid*), which was first isolated in the 1930s and first used as an anti-inflammatory agent in 1948 by Dr. Philip Hench, a rheumatologist at the Mayo Clinic. He administered cortisone (an extract of the adrenal gland), or "Compound E" as it was then called, to tamp down a patient's chronic inflammation, combining it with a course of morphine or other opiates to control the pain. Hench and Dr. Edward Kendall, a hormone chemist, had extracted and purified Compound E (which came from cow adrenal glands) over a two-year period. It was hailed as a miracle—and it was. Patients were able to walk for the first time in years after getting a single cortisone injection. For their efforts in ingeniously curing generations of severe pain and disabling disease, the two men received the Nobel Prize for Physiology or Medicine in 1950.

Today, we use chemically made or synthetic cortisone, but history has not been kind to cortisone in either form. The side effects are legendary: high blood sugars (diabetes), thinning of and damage to the skin, easy bruising, blanching of bone, bone loss (osteoporosis), bloating, increased appetite ... I saw mice in a lab fatten up so much after cortisone shots that they had problems scurrying around their cages and looked like pears with legs. Some patients have even suffered from immunosuppression. Treating these side effects requires the cessation of cortisone treatment, which leads to RA relapse.

These unfortunate side effects went unrecorded for years. Some of the reason is surely because the effects were so numerous and varied, so it took a while to link them to the cause. Some of the reason can be attributed to the fact that cortisone was so effective and ameliorating of pain—and so immediate in people who were suffering—that "consequences be damned." It is easy for me to understand why: I have films of patients who were unable to walk before an injection of the cortisone and then after the injection miraculously run up and down stairs, free of pain. Some of the reason for the cavalier attitude with corticosteroids was that the biochemistry of inflammation was not understood when Hench and Kendall did their work. That understanding was in place in the 1960s when modern science found a different approach: nonsteroidal anti-inflammatory drugs, or NSAIDs.

You know the first NSAID: aspirin. It was invented in 1897. The rest you might have heard of generically like ibuprofen, naproxen, diclofenac, celecoxib, mefenamic acid, etoricoxib, and indomethacin.[2] NSAIDs are the most common pain medications in the world, most prescribed anti-inflammatory medications for treating RA, and sufficient for most people's control of inflammation. They are a trillion-dollar market all over the world. Like cortisone, NSAIDs also have side effects; they are tough on the kidneys, raise your blood pressure, and can even cause heart attacks if abused. In fact, the first anti-inflammatory drug, phenylbutazone, was eventually removed from the market because of its toxic effects on bone marrow in some people. I have an ashtray that my father used in the 1950s with a phenylbutazone advertisement on the base. Two early losers, smoking and a new drug that caused problems were evident in our living room. But every drug has side effects and is a trade-off—with the good effects, you can get something bad in return, just not as bad as they are with cortisone.

Not that cortisone and its chemical relatives have gone away. Hardly. While rarely used for long-term treatment because of those side effects, they remain important anti-inflammatories to treat profound inflammation and severe flares of rheumatoid arthritis, lupus, and other diseases that require an immediate resolution. Other corticosteroids are used to relieve swelling, redness, and other inflammation, like the powerful dexamethasone mentioned before and used to combat the effects of COVID-19 in the lung.

---

[2] I got to see how indomethacin worked firsthand, when I was in high school in the early 1960s. I had a summer job in the research institute at the pharmaceutical company Merck. In the lab tests, rats with an experimental form of RA were divided into two groups. One rat was injected with cortisone, the other got a new nonsteroidal synthetic, which eventually became known as indomethacin, a wonderful pain reliever and anti-inflammatory agent as this new class of anti-inflammatory agents was born.

DR. BOB SAYS

Corticosteroids like cortisone and its chemical relatives provide miraculous immediate relief from pain and inflammation, but they have serious side effects when taken long-term, including weight gain and immunosuppression. Nonsteroidal drugs (meaning not related to cortisone and its chemical relatives) are widely used and extremely useful against inflammation. They take away pain and swelling and are relatively safe when taken in moderation, but like all drugs, especially when not taken in moderation, they too have drawbacks, which is why they are not long-term solutions to pain either.

Here's another rub when it comes to cortisone: immunosuppression. When you're talking about immune modulation, you're talking about immunosuppression or suppression of the body's immune system and its ability to fight infections and other diseases. Trying to control the immune system by turning it down, as we learned in the last chapter, can result in increased morbidity and even mortality in patients who take these drugs, especially over time. In other words, you could die from the smallest of invasions. Remember what happens in HIV patients: helper T cells (CD4) are completely obliterated. Patients can die from innocuous organisms like bread mold or a bacillus that lives on the skin and would be harmless to people with healthy immune systems. Immunosuppression is something your doctor can modify and judiciously monitor, and doctors routinely do in the case of the autoimmune diseases we see, but it is a problem for patients on these drugs.

But perhaps the biggest drawback to cortisone and NSAIDs is that they are not long-term solutions. They require daily doses to be effective and don't actually target what causes the inflammation, just the inflammation itself. When modern medicine started using corticosteroids and nonsteroid treatments to fight this fire, there was no alternative—no idea that there might be a way to harness the immune system and create biologicals that would turn this or that cytokine off relieving the patient of inflammation and sometimes organ destruction. Eventually, scientists began to wonder, *Could there be a better way?*

As with all things scientific, as Louis Pasteur said, "chance favors the prepared mind." Enter monoclonal antibodies.

NEXT GEN FIREFIGHTERS: MONOCLONAL ANTIBODIES

Antibodies are proteins naturally produced by plasma cells in your immune system that respond to inflammatory invasions by criminal antigens and pathogens and destroy them. They are analogous to handcuffs for your first responders because they wrap around the criminal invader and allow it to be engulfed by neutrophils—those white blood cell germ eaters and paddy wagons—and sent to the Alcatraz of your body, the spleen, or your lymph node for destruction. Within our blood there is an antibody repertoire, like sheet music, that is specific and efficient. Most of these antibodies are polyclonal (meaning they are produced by different immune cells) that are directed to specific antigens based on immune genetics (meaning they have their own specific structure and are "called up" from plasma cells to attach to those antigens). While polyclonal antibodies are directed to a specific antigen, they bind themselves to different epitopes or parts of the antigen.

Monoclonal antibodies are much more than just handcuffs: They are your immune system's natural equivalent of a guided missile. They are produced by a single clone of plasma cells and target one specific antigen and epitope. Today, these guided missiles have been engineered in a lab, each one an identical copy of the missile designed to bond to one specific antigen and to mimic or enhance the body's natural immune response against an invader, be it cancer or COVID-19, each providing molecular therapies against their cytokines and chemokines.[3]

Engineering "designer" monoclonal antibodies are something Hench and Kendall could only have dreamed of in 1948, and even if they did dream, the process of cultivating plasma cells that produce antibodies was hard and inefficient. Scientists didn't find another way forward until 1974 when Georges J. F. Köhler and César Milstein developed a technique called *hybridoma generation*. In this technique, *hybridoma cells*—a fusion of B cells and myeloma cells or malignancies from human blood—create an antigen-specific monoclonal antibody.

Hybridoma generation was a clever fusing of a malignant clone of cells with B cells that could proliferate to produce one benign collection of cells that made huge amounts of specific antibody. Most monoclonal antibodies produced in great amounts in patients are the result of this myeloma, a cancer of the blood; monoclonal antibodies in hybridoma generation are made from a clone of malignant plasma cells that is not cancerous. This technique led to their discovery of a principle for the production of monoclonal antibodies to control the immune system, for which they were awarded the Nobel Prize in Physiology or Medicine in 1984. The first monoclonal antibody, derived from a single B cell, was developed soon after Köhler and Milstein's discovery and researchers started producing and testing different monoclonal antibodies readily and efficiently in mice or other animals using hybridoma generation, including the lab I worked in.

Here's how hybridoma generation worked. A mouse was immunized against a specific antigen, so that mouse would produce antibodies in response to that antigen. We then took the B lymphocytes (white blood cells) the mouse produced from its spleen

---

[3] Monoclonal therapy of COVID-19 is available for acute illness. It blocks the binding of the virus to the specific receptors needed for ingestion in cells. Some combined monoclonals from companies like Regeneron are used as an effective therapy.

and fused them (chemically or through a virus method) with the myeloma cells from a patient, which had been grown in the lab. (They are not hard to grow, because cancer cells like to proliferate, even in a test tube.) Once this hybridoma or single clone of cells was generated, it was screened to see if the specific antibody was made. If it was, using a very specialized procedure using a variety of chemical methods to eliminate all nonspecific antibodies, the cells multiplied in the abdomen of the mouse and voilà! A single clone of cells called a hybridoma successfully produced a few milliliters of a single monoclonal antibody in the mouse's belly. Once that single monoclonal antibody was produced, the next step was industrial production. because each human patient needs varying amounts of it for treatment, and there are only so many milliliters available from the mouse belly.

Of course, as you know now, the human immune system would reject anything that it considered foreign, including a protein from a mouse cell. So, using techniques from molecular biology, we placed human genes inside the mouse in place of the mouse's genes (in their B cells in particular) to generate human monoclonal antibodies in mice that we as humans would not reject. In other words, the human immune system would make human anti-mouse antibody. (You might want to read that sentence again). This anti-mouse antibody quickly neutralized the presence of the mouse antibody that was being used to attack the human T cells and over time rendered it useless. The result was the ability to develop antibodies that target just about any antigen.

We called these mouse heroes "humanized mice," not because they have the ability to talk or read (as many of my colleagues like to joke), but because the process of implanting human genes into a mouse or any animal to produce an antibody human won't reject is called humanization. Today, the method of production uses cultured cells from a Chinese hamster ovary or similar animal, but we are striving to move beyond the need for humanization and get these antibodies to develop in something more humane like yeast, which also grows a lot faster than cells from a hamster.

It took until 1986 for all this to come together, human trials to be completed, and the Food and Drug Administration (FDA) to approve the first monoclonal antibody for clinical use: muromonab-CD3, which prevented kidney (and other organ) transplant rejection. Muromonab-CD3 is primitive by today's standards but was remarkable then. It targeted the CD3 receptors of T lymphocyte cells (CD3 is a general marker for T cells), binding itself to the surface of those cells and preventing them from communicating with your natural killer T cells and telling them that the transplanted kidney was a foreign invader that must be attacked and destroyed.

While there were side effects, including reducing the body's ability to fight infections, muromonab-CD3 ushered in a whole new era of immunotherapeutic drugs that have saved millions of lives. They are revolutionizing medicine worldwide, especially when it comes to the RA from which Sam and so many others suffer.

Consider Juanita, who had none of the advantages of Sam growing up. She arrived at my clinic from a village in Ecuador with a very progressive case of RA. Juanita was in incredible pain. Her hands and feet were greatly deformed. She could barely walk or grip even a pencil. At 40, the same age as Sam in 2011, Juanita looked like she was 80. That's because there was no modern RA treatment available in her village. She had only the occasional cortisone shot and a series of cortisone pills to help her manage, which she took only intermittently because of the cost. Our initial treatment tapered her off the cortisone (so that her system would not be shocked by the rapid decline of the drug). We then did an assessment of her bones, blood tests, and some of the RA-specific assays. But when it came to treatment, we skipped right over NSAIDs and went right to fighting her inflammation with biologicals engineered from monoclonal antibodies, specifically ones targeting tumor necrosis factor (TNF), an inflammatory cytokine antigen, which was the source of her and most RA patients' inflammation and pain (as well as the destruction of her joints).

TNF is a host defense molecule that acts as one of your immune system's most important danger detection systems. One of the first cytokines that appear in the blood after an injury or stress, it sounds an alarm within minutes.[4] Dr. Anthony Cerami, a Rockefeller University investigator, was the first person I knew who had the idea that bacterial sepsis (infection of the blood with possible shock and death) could be treated by blocking TNF. Dr. Ravinder Maini (an emeritus professor at Imperial College London) and Dr. Mark Feldman (today the head of Oxford's Kennedy Institute of Rheumatology) took the next step and conducted the first clinical trial of TNF blockade in any disease apart from sepsis by using a kind of micro sponge made in the lab (etanercept). The TNF blockade result was a rheumatologic revelation and a revolution, taking their principles of removing TNF to a new level. Corticosteroids could take a backseat with this development of a monoclonal antibody missile targeting TNF and inhibiting it in patients with severe RA.

The result today is that there are many monoclonal antibodies directed against TNF to treat RA and other diseases. The first, etanercept (sold under the name Enbrel), was approved in 1998. Others like adalimumab (sold under the name Humira starting in 2002) followed. Interestingly, the monoclonal antibody that became etanercept was discovered when another drug was being used in England to treat inflammatory bowel disease. During the therapy, the doctors noticed that the patients also had complete resolution of their arthritis. They decided to start using the drug for patients with RA—clearly an example of chance favoring a prepared mind!—and found it so effective against the TNF cytokines that researchers decided to develop a monoclonal antibody against TNF. Thus, a generation of biologicals for RA was born.[5]

---

[4] Other cytokines we call pro-inflammatory, such as interleukin 1 or interleukin 6, appear later, but there is evidence that their appearance usually follows the prior release of TNF.

[5] Dr. Cerami today has a patent on the anti-TNF monoclonal antibody that has been approved by the FDA for the treatment of RA as well as Crohn's disease, continuing the connection found in England.

Like any treatment, inhibition of cytokines has its trade-offs. Patients must be tested for hepatitis as well as TB before going on these drugs, because TB or hepatitis can be reactivated if those bugs are nesting somewhere in your body. In addition, a severe bacterial infection of a joint or skin can be deadly if the anti-TNF is not discontinued. But for most patients like Juanita and Sam, these were minor considerations. Biologicals may not have been a cure for their RA but were just as good as one because they stopped the progression of the disease in their joints and relieved their pain and inflammation without a daily course of corticosteroids or cortisone.

Soon after our treatment of Juanita, she had no new erosions, gained weight, felt better, and looked like a different person. All because her TNF cytokine was lowered. This is immunotherapy at its best, just decades after the research started.

DR. BOB SAYS

Monoclonal antibodies can be used against bad cells like cancers, against allergic cells in certain diseases, and even to help regulate things like bone growth in people with osteoporosis. The possibilities are endless. Using monoclonal antibodies against cytokines—the communication molecules of your immune system—has a major clinical effect on chronic inflammatory diseases. When you get rid of the cytokine, you cure patients without harm. The only problem is the immunosuppressive effect of the cytokine blocker, which can reactivate infections and propagate some that have just begun.

THE FUTURE OF BIOLOGICALS

Since the arrival of muromonab-CD3, more than 100 monoclonal antibodies have been approved to treat many diseases beyond RA, and many more are in clinical trials. Monoclonal antibody therapy is used to treat conditions like systemic lupus, inflammatory bowel disease, Crohn's disease, ulcerative colitis, psoriatic arthritis, psoriasis, ankylosing spondylitis, juvenile RA, and many diseases you probably have never heard of and hopefully never will need to. But if you are a patient or know someone with any of those diseases, you understand the biological revolution and what it means to fight fire with fire.

There are biologicals targeting insulin and thyroid receptors, stimulating or inhibiting the actions of organs or to turn off cells that make antibodies themselves. Some are being used to attack specific pain receptors and stop pain. Some scientists are using fragments of monoclonal antibodies like smart bombs, as opposed to missiles, to minimize unnecessary casualties called targeted immunotherapy. We can also use biologicals to limit white cells and endothelial cells (those cells on the surface of blood vessels)—sticky molecules that have proven to be useful in the dissection of the mechanisms of inflammation. This allows us to develop new drugs to treat patients and to understand diseases that were thought to be inflammatory but are not.

Simply put, immunity in the face of antigens and more has never looked stronger with these guided missiles coming of age. For example, in the case of lupus, the monoclonal antibody known as belimumab became the first to attack *B lymphocyte stimulating factor*. It seems that in lupus, the B lymphocytes are stimulated to become outlaw producers of autoantibodies by a trigger that allows the cells to break tolerance. Until the discovery of belimumab in 2001, doctors had no treatment for this disease other than corticosteroids and chemotherapeutic agents.

Or consider monoclonal antibodies against COVID-19. When President Trump contracted the virus, they rushed him to Bethesda Naval Hospital for treatment, where he was given a monoclonal antibody against the viral spike protein along with large doses of dexamethasone. While the data was new, those of us treating COVID-19 patients on the frontline knew that the monoclonal antibody along with dexamethasone had an incredibly good chance of success in controlling the acute COVID-19 infectious process. While not effective with everyone, it worked for the president, and since then more monoclonal antibodies have been derived that react with the spike protein and continued to be used for those infected early in the ER and those in the MICU who are acutely ill.[6] Of course, the variants of the spike protein from the COVID-19 virus could become resistant to the monoclonal antibody developed for the initial strain, but our advancements in this area allow us to isolate the variant's spike protein and make new monoclonal antibody missiles to break through its adaptive defenses.

When I think of all we have covered, I am grateful not only to the researchers but to my, and countless other, lab mice who sacrificed their lives to produce the hybridomas that started the monoclonal antibody revolution—a revolution that is continuing in so many ways. The most exciting of which are in the world of cancer.

FIGHTING THE FIRE OF CANCER: CHECKPOINT THERAPY AND MORE

What happens when you connect the dots through all we have covered in this and the previous chapter and use it to target cancer? If you're James Allison and Tasuku Honjo, you develop immune

---

[6] Early in the COVID-19 pandemic, we were all using convalescent serum as a research tool. Convalescent serum was extracted from patients who were infected with the virus, and who had high titers of anti-COVID-19 antibody. It is curious that this polyclonal antibody obtained from patients postinfection was very inconsistent, because not everybody made large amounts of polyclonal antibody to the virus. The reason for this inconsistency with regard to viral infection is probably based on everyone's genetic response. The convalescence sera obtained from a patient who had high titers of the antibodies that neutralize the virus did work to control serious disease in some patients. However, the polyclonal antibody had to be obtained from the patient's plasma, purified, and then reinfused into another patient. From this description, you can see how wonderful a monoclonal antibody directed against a specific antigen like a spike protein from a coronavirus would be extremely useful. In President Trump and many others, it was.

checkpoint therapy—an immunotherapy that channels the energy the immune system might put into autoimmune anarchy to attack cancer cells. In other words, they found a way to cure certain cancers immunologically. For this discovery, Allison and Honjo were awarded the 2018 Nobel Prize in Medicine, and it is every bit as deserving and amazing as it sounds.

In their crafty criminal states, tumors like melanoma, colon, lung, liver, and almost any other you can think of are sophisticated enough to get around the immune system by blocking T cells with specific protein molecules—a kind of protective barrier to T cell action—which mediate tumor immunity. Cells that are transplanted into us that are foreign are rejected immediately, largely as a result of the MHC-directed T cells that control the appearance of foreign tissues. The problem with cancer is that T lymphocytes become anergic (lose their immune potency) or they are deleted when in the company of a tumor, preventing a reaction that would rid the body of the tumor. This is why tumors are like an autonomous zone that exist in some cities, Native American reservations, or even a cult controlling its compound by enforcing its own laws and refusing entry to "outsider" first responders; they are singularly able to control the local T cell response by secreting cytokines like IL-10 or TGF-beta and stop the T cells from getting in. Your first responders are essentially stuck on the outside of the compound, unable to breach the barrier.

Allison and Honjo's checkpoint therapy target regulatory pathways in T cells to enhance antitumor immune responses. The name comes from the checkpoint protein they studied, CTLA-4, which forms a barrier around the tumor. The therapy they derived is not a chemical but a biological—an engineered monoclonal antibody that attacks the CTLA-4 proteins that protect the tumor. That's right: Instead of attacking the tumor, checkpoint attacks this protective network and removes it with antibodies against these protective antigens that belong to the tumor. It's like an episode of *Star Trek* in which the crew finds a way to take the enemy's shields down, and the captain of the *Enterprise* says,

"Fire at will!" In this case, the photon torpedoes are our natural killer T cells.

> ### DR. BOB SAYS
>
> The immune system recognizes patterns and receptors. We can fool the immune system to attack solid tumors by removing their protective coating, or we can remove T cells and re-educate them to attack blood malignancies.

There is an ongoing effort to identify predictive biomarkers for immune checkpoint therapies, and even a combination of checkpoint therapy and standard chemotherapy for melanomas and tumors of many organs, including the pancreas, one of the deadliest cancers. Checkpoint therapy is also being used to shrink tumors so they can be removed later surgically without damaging too much of the organ.

In addition to checkpoint, we also now have CAR T cell therapy or "chimeric antigen receptor T cell therapy," which removes the T cells from cancer patients and trains them in the laboratory to find and destroy any of your cancer cells directly. Most of the time, T cells become activated when the tumor antigens are recognized, leading to the T cell's ability to attack and destroy the cells that express the relevant antigens. CAR T-cell therapy, sometimes called cell-based gene therapy, alters the genes inside of T cells to treat a cancer more efficiently. It effectively "personalizes" the therapy based on the genomic sequencing of each person's cancer cells to identify the specific mutations of genes that the tumor has, making the T cells more efficient at attacking cancers with different receptors on their surfaces. The trained T cells are then injected back into the patient. Amazingly, the data shows that tumors can be completely obliterated using this personalized treatment, making CAR T cell therapy a breakthrough for nonsolid tumors or those of the blood, like leukemia or lymphoma.

To understand even a part of this is to be on the cusp of the medical revolution we are experiencing when it comes to boosting the immune system from the outside and being immunity strong. This is truly us helping our biological soul help us live longer and may eventually even replace a treatment that is several hundred years old to prevent modern diseases: the vaccine.

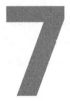

7 Vaccines in the Age of COVID-19

Think back to Chapter 1 and Greg, a healthy young man whose COVID-19 infection had him suffering from a "whiteout" in both his lungs caused by a cytokine storm in which his immune system was suddenly attacking his organs. Placed on a ventilator, Greg beat the odds and barely survived. A year later, if Greg had received any of the three COVID-19 vaccines widely available in the United States at the time, there is almost no chance he would have ended up in the hospital from his infection, let alone faced death—even if he contracted a breakthrough variant of COVID-19. Millions no longer grace our tables because of the horror of COVID-19 but hundreds of millions are still with us because they either were immune, asymptomatic, or never faced any severe acute symptoms from an infection because of those vaccines. From a medical perspective, it is awe-inspiring.

Before we continue, in the interest of transparency, let me be clear where I am coming from: I am a fan of vaccines, get them myself, administer them, and think they are almost always better than the alternative of getting what you're being vaccinated against. I voted yes when the leadership of my hospital decided to mandate the annual flu injection or risk termination. I stated many times in interviews that I believe all first responders should be fully vaccinated to avoid catastrophic infection to which they are exposed daily. Because of the awful burden on our society, I think we should also mandate COVID-19 and flu vaccines for those who work directly with people and continue to do so (with limited exceptions, including religious objections).

It is my greatest hope that vaccines be widely and easily available to every person living in our country. I also think all vaccines, not just those for public health emergencies, must remain free or so inexpensive that everyone can afford them, and we need ongoing community access, education, and mobilization around them. Sadly, that is not the case overall. Their availability around the world remains a problem, largely because technology and availability are not equal in rich and poor countries. But even if it were, vaccine hesitancy would be an issue.

In April 2021, the United States passed 50 percent of the eligible population fully vaccinated against COVID-19, but the rate of vaccination had slowed, making herd immunity or having 70 to 80 percent of the population vaccinated or immune to the disease unlikely. Eligibility and access were major culprits in the slowing of vaccination, but most of us also learned a term during this time: "vaccine hesitancy." The reasons for vaccine hesitancy are complex. Many people were not against the COVID-19 vaccine but maybe needed an incentive (a free amusement park ride, a lottery ticket, or in some cases, a free beer) or were more what we might call "vaccine maybe"—people like pregnant women and others simply waiting for more data and research to be convinced. But media stories tended to focus on what we might call "vaccine no"—outright resistance to the COVID-19 vaccine tied to political beliefs (e.g., white male conservatives being the most resistant), religious objections, or the troubling story of the Tuskegee Study that led to many Black people's mistrust of the medical system.

Wild conspiracy theories passing as "news" on social media surrounding the rollout of COVID-19 vaccines and vaccines in general only fueled vaccine resistance. This "news" has been misleading, highly exaggerated, or patently false, making the subject of vaccines polarizing for reasons that are anything but scientific. In addition, many stories from well-respected sources focus on the negative instead of the good vaccines do. After all, "Person Dies from Vaccine" or "People Resist Vaccination" is much more powerful clickbait than "Nothing Bad Happens because of Vaccinations." A 2021 NPR analysis that found that "articles connecting vaccines and death have been among the most highly engaged with content online this year, going viral in a way that could hinder people's ability to judge the true risk in getting a shot." These stories fuel our emotions, and emotions more than science or facts rule our behavior. They are also fueling the supposed facts behind the growing anti-vaccine or anti-vaxxer movement, which cites an autism-vaccine link that is worthless, medically and otherwise.

This link can be directly traced to a now thoroughly and completely discredited paper in the medical journal *Lancet* by Andrew Wakefield in 1998. In it, Wakefield claimed that pediatric immunizations for measles, mumps, and rubella caused autism. His allegations were subsequently disproved, and the paper withdrawn. (Wakefield was struck from the medical register in his native England, which is why I don't even call him a doctor.) You by now know the immune system is not innocent in causing neurodegenerative and behavioral diseases, and that vaccines are not perfect. But vaccination is not the cause of autism, full stop, and is essential to the health of our immune systems.

Still, I can throw that explanation and all the science I have at unvaccinated people, and I would likely not sway them, because we are all less likely to be swayed by facts than our relationships—by people we know, look like us, truly connect with, or who align with our beliefs. Shaming people who are hesitant is no way to overcome this distrust. Neither are government mandates that are troubling, legally dubious, and even more divisive. I also can't solve for emotions or politics in this book.

So, what to do?

COVID-19, like influenza and many other illnesses, will be endemic (meaning commonly found) and with us forever. They will change and adapt, and we will likely need annual vaccinations to cover all the variants that some viruses—even those we thought eradicated—become. That, you know now, is what viruses do; they jump species, change, adapt, and evolve. This chapter builds on that knowledge you have and offers a bit of history and discussion of how vaccines work, how they deliver immunity or work to strengthen your immune system, and a little understanding of the marvel that was the COVID-19 response by answering the following questions:

- What are vaccines and where did they originate?
- How are vaccines developed?
- What are the different kinds of vaccines?
- What is a booster shot?
- What are adjuvants? Aren't they dangerous?
- There *are* side effects to vaccines—isn't that bad?
- Why do we still fear vaccines?

While you don't know me, we've spent some time together now. Maybe by answering these questions, I can help you or someone you know evolve your perspective on vaccines.

WHAT ARE VACCINES AND WHERE DID THEY ORIGINATE?

A vaccine is medicine that trains your body to fight foreign invasions and, in many cases, provides acquired immunity to the invader. All vaccines begin with an exposure to a virus or pathogen to trigger a strong cellular immune response that involves your MHC class I natural killer T cells. They learn to respond to that viral infection and eliminate it.

Vaccines have been with us for more than 200 years and no advance in public health short of sanitation has been more important. Both control infections, the leading causes of death in the world. The origin of the word vaccine comes from *vacca*, the Latin word for a cow. That's because the vaccination story begins with Edward Jenner, an English country doctor who used a live but weakened or attenuated foreign antigen found in the exudate (pus) from a pustule of cowpox and injected it into a boy to create a state of immune protection against the smallpox virus. The inoculation worked. In 1880, Louis Pasteur built on the work of Jenner when he realized old chicken cholera germs could not transmit the disease and used them to develop a lab-created vaccine to inoculate chickens against the disease. He later created animal vaccines against rabies and anthrax.

Jenner's and Pasteur's monumental work using weakened or attenuated organisms to create a state of immune protection is the foundation for the *live-attenuated vaccines* we are familiar with today. The principles of this vaccination depend on using these organisms—or, more recently, parts of the organism—to produce an immune response. Adaptive and cellular immunity to specific infections can be achieved by deliberately causing that infection with an unmodified infectious agent like Jenner did with smallpox.

DR. BOB SAYS

Vaccines are a major public health benefit and true scientific marvels that have been with us for more than a century. Safe and cheap, they have been proven effective in preventing or mitigating the effects of many illnesses and saving lives.

HOW ARE VACCINES DEVELOPED?

Consider the brilliance of those early scientists who developed protective measures called vaccines before there was any knowledge about antibodies or cellular response or that there was even something called an immune system. Today, technology has scaled the work of Pasteur, allowing vaccines to be developed safely and quickly using the organism's genes to make them in a lab in "high tech" time. Note, when I say quickly, I do not mean the development of vaccines; I mean the production. Vaccine development ordinarily takes 10 to 15 years and involves many years of expensive and in-depth research, testing, and clinical trials to ensure three things before being established as preventive for disease:

1. The vaccine must be deemed safe, because any low level of toxicity to the patient is not acceptable.
2. The vaccine must be efficient and protect most people who get it.
3. The vaccine must offer long-term, if not permanent, immunity, with continuing strength in the neutralizing antibody and robust cellular response.

That's why, like all medications, all vaccines—even those for COVID-19's accelerated timetable—must complete a three-phase human process.

- Phase 1: Ensure the immune response occurs when the vaccine is administered. This is the most rudimentary aspect of the development phase and primarily exists for safety and to establish dosage.
- Phase 2: Expanded trials in which a potential vaccine is given to hundreds of people to see if the vaccine stimulates the immune system, agrees with people, and has any toxic effects. Ideally, this group includes people of all ages, sexes, races, ethnicities, and from all parts of any country.
- Phase 3: The "efficacy trial," in which the vaccine is given to thousands and tens of thousands of people (again ideally covering all those groups listed in phase two) to see how many become infected compared with people who get a placebo or sugar injection. This phase determines whether the vaccine truly protects against the infection and can proceed to review and authorization.

Authorization starts with an independent committee within each company, then the oversight committee of the FDA, followed by the FDA advisory committee, which includes epidemiologists, infectious disease experts, general medicine practitioners, statisticians, and even some laypeople. While the FDA review is going on, a company can seek an emergency-use authorization to speed distribution, as was the case with COVID-19 as the pandemic meant every human on the planet needed a dose. Once everything is approved, vaccine production and distribution begins.

As I said before, the COVID-19 vaccine development was a marvel, particularly as so many companies succeeded so quickly. But we should have had some hope: Today, many vaccines are so safe, abundant, and long-lasting that they are administered to the most vulnerable among us: infants and young children, pregnant women, and the elderly. As a result, polio, tetanus, hepatitis A and B, measles, rubella, mumps, chicken pox, pertussis or whooping cough, diphtheria, and *Haemophilus influenzae type b*, or Hib, have been controlled in most people who get the vaccines. And while it took some time since Jenner's day, smallpox was eradicated globally in 1980, one of public health's greatest triumphs.

DR. BOB SAYS

It takes many steps to have a vaccine approved, even on an emergency basis. Advisory councils are very tough and spend days and weeks going over data before debating it and ensuring it is reliable and convincing and the vaccine is safe.

WHAT ARE THE DIFFERENT KINDS OF VACCINES?

Until COVID-19, the most common vaccines were those *live-attenuated vaccines* from live organisms that are grown until they are weakened and no longer infect humans in an efficient manner.

These are then injected into humans (or sprayed into noses as is the case with the nasal flu vaccine) to stimulate immunity, not the disease. Live-attenuated vaccines are extremely effective at what they target. They have eliminated polio in most countries and control the scourge of measles, mumps, rubella, varicella, and pertussis (whooping cough).

There are some limitations to live-attenuated vaccines. They are not always suited to combating mutations of a disease. They also must be kept cold and deteriorate when taken from storage. So, for example, while the measles vaccine is highly effective, it is unstable in warm climates and difficult to use in tropical developing countries. This keeps infant deaths from the disease in these countries at an unacceptable high. In addition, while live-attenuated vaccines are effective, getting the organisms for these vaccines has not always been easy and is time-consuming. Thus, science started looking for another way, and the first COVID-19 vaccines put those approaches on display.

First up was the first widespread use of two *genetic vaccines*. These vaccines inject the coronavirus's own messenger RNA or selective RNA genes to make the immune system believe that the virus has infected the cells, provoking an immune response. One of the companies producing this vaccine, the pharmaceutical giant Pfizer, partnered with BioNTech, a small German company that was working on cancer vaccines, to design it. BioNTech tested 20 different stretches of mRNA out of 33,000 genes to find the portions of the genome that code for the COVID-19 spike protein, the most immunogenic of the proteins from the virus to which the immune system reacts and the protein with which the virus attaches to specific receptors in the nose, eyes, throat and of course the lung, heart, and brain.

Injection of nucleic acids like DNA or RNA was not new to research labs and vaccine makers. DNA from influenza virus has been able to prevent infections in mice after injection. But a human genetic vaccine had not arrived when COVID-19 hit, so no one thought that a genetic vaccine would be the first or most successful vaccine to reach the market. A big reason for this delay was that scientists had to make sure dendritic cells—part of your immune system's central command team in your innate response—could take up the mRNA in the vaccine and present the spike protein to our T lymphocytes (and subsequently B cells) to allow our immune system's adaptive response to produce the antibody.[1]

Once they solved getting the dendritic cell issue, genetic vaccines faced another problem. No, not any irrational fear about genetic materials being injected into you. Messenger RNA enters the cytoplasm of the cell that manufactures the spike protein. It never gets into the nucleus where DNA is located. Nothing is programmed, hijacked, or mutated. The problem was logistics. Genetic or mRNA vaccines require extreme refrigeration, well below the temperatures needed for live-attenuated vaccines. This sensitivity comes from the very nature of RNA, which is a delicate molecule and susceptible to heat and bodily enzymes. The novel creation of a fat-covered nanoparticle to deliver this vaccine to the cells once in the body saved the day. An NPR story compared the RNA to the chocolate inside an M&M: With heat, the chocolate melts in your hand, but with the sugar coating it melts in your mouth—the nanoparticle was the "candy shell" that delivered mRNA's "chocolate" to your immune system before it "melted."

Once these internal and external logistics problems were solved, clinical trials proceeded with unprecedented speed. Pfizer's

---

[1] The story of vaccines in my professional life dates back to when I entered medicine. I have bad memories of a 16-year-old girl at the Rockefeller University research hospital from whom we obtained measles antibodies on a biweekly basis. She had developed measles brain disease at a young age, a condition wherein she continuously shed measles virus and went into a vegetative state because she did not get the measles vaccine when she was young. She became a living laboratory who supported researchers with volumes of sera and cells to study viruses and the many ways the immune system might act to prevent them from taking hold. This same lab was where my friend, the late Nobel laureate Dr. Ralph Steinman, discovered dendritic cells, which would many years later be the key in understanding the innate immune system's efficacy and the COVID-19 vaccines' effectiveness.

mRNA vaccine, followed by Moderna's, finished their phase three trials in record time, achieving 90 percent efficacy after testing some 50,000 plus individuals, and genetic vaccines were approved for emergency use around the world. While these vaccines need a second shot in most people to be completely effective and will likely need booster vaccines because of the variants of COVID-19, those variants will only require genetic tinkering with the existing vaccine, not the development of a whole new vaccine.

The third COVID-19 vaccine approved for use in the United States, Janssen (Johnson & Johnson), was a *viral vector vaccine*. Before COVID-19, viral vector technology had been used to fight Ebola outbreaks by modifying an innocuous version of one virus (which does not sicken the host) to attack another by delivering its genes into cells and provoke an immune response. In the Johnson & Johnson vaccine, you will see this innocuous virus listed as the main ingredient: *recombinant, replication-incompetent adenovirus type 26 expressing the SARS-CoV-2 spike protein.*[2] While viral vector vaccines had less effectiveness than genetic vaccines at stopping COVID-19 infections completely, they have been as incredible at stopping severe infections and death. And in good news for warmer climates, these vaccines do not need to be refrigerated.

The list of COVID-19 vaccines will surely be longer by the time you read this and administered in even more ways. As I write, nearly 300 vaccines were being developed and more than 90 of those in various stages of testing. For those people with trypanophobia (fear of injections or needles), two of the vaccines being developed are oral and seven are nasal. These vaccines include an entirely different kind of vaccine: the *protein subunit* or *acellular vaccine*.

---

[2] The vaccine from AstraZeneca in Oxford, England, which started the search for a vaccine before COVID-19 was declared pandemic and was prepared to move forward quicker than any of the other vaccines, is also a viral vector vaccine. Unfortunately, several missteps by the company surrounding its data and dealing with side effects led to suspicion about the vaccine and its approval lagged behind the others in the United States and was halted in others.

Unlike live-attenuated vaccines, which use a whole weakened organism, subunit vaccines use purified specific fragments of the virus or bacterium's protein to provoke an immune response. In the case of COVID-19, the vaccine would likely use the virus's specific spike protein fragment to produce immunity. The best part of these vaccines is they have been well tolerated by people with weak immune systems. The trade-off of this tolerance is their strength: subunit vaccines can require boosters to be effective.

The only kind of vaccine not being developed for COVID-19 that exists for other diseases is the *toxoid vaccine*. Toxoid vaccines are chemically treated toxins from bacteria like tetanus toxin, diphtheria toxin, and botulism toxin. These toxins are heat treated or chemically inactivated with formaldehyde, but their antigenicity is preserved so that your immune system will react and prevent you from getting these terrible illnesses.

DR. BOB SAYS

Vaccines are amazingly effective ways to keep your immune system strong. Molecular science now allows us to develop genetic vaccines that include the nucleic acids of the offending criminals, eliminating any fear about having a weak bug injected into you.

WHAT IS A BOOSTER SHOT?

Even when a vaccine is effective, it may need adjustments. For example, Hib (*Haemophilus influenzae B*), a leading cause of bacterial meningitis in children, was reformulated two years after it arrived to be more effective in children under 18 months. On the flip side, the pertussis vaccine was incredibly effective but was shown to have some side effects and allergic reactions that were more than rare. Its reformulation avoided those effects but made the vaccine less effective, leading to outbreaks in the twenty-first century for the first time since the 1940s. That led to a recommended Tdap vaccine booster (which also includes diphtheria and tetanus) for children 11 or 12 years old.

As I said before, the strong cellular responses to vaccines involve your MHC class I natural killer T cells that respond to a viral infection. If that cellular response and/or the antibody weakens over time, a booster shot may be needed. In the case of influenza and infections like COVID-19, there are so many variants and mutations that a yearly vaccine is (or likely will be) needed as a boost.

Influenza changes its proverbial coat each year; actually, it wears many constantly changing coats (i.e., strains) of varying degrees of deadliness. The deadliest was the Spanish flu or 1918 influenza pandemic. An H1N1 influenza virus with avian genes, it eventually killed 3 percent of the U.S. population alone (638,000 people) and reduced life expectancy in the country by 12 years. Unfortunately, there were no flu vaccines back then—influenza was only isolated as a virus in 1933 and a vaccine was not available until after World War II, though not for the Spanish flu. Even with the number of flu vaccines today, the Spanish flu's coat-changing descendants avoid our defenses and kill millions when they do. In fact, many scientists believe the Spanish flu never went away and just continues to adapt, evolve, and jump species. That's what happens when an infection becomes endemic and variable.

We were approaching a Spanish flu number of fatalities for COVID-19 and facing similar concerns about the future when the first vaccines appeared. While these emergency-use COVID-19 vaccines were nearly perfect at preventing severe illness and death, they were less effective at preventing COVID-19. But they were still more effective than the shingles vaccine (about 50 percent effective at preventing the disease for five years) or the flu vaccine (40 to 60 percent effective each year). Still, unless you have an allergy or autoimmune condition that would cause an adverse reaction, getting these shots and possibly avoiding the disease is much better than the alternative despite the rare side effects we will cover shortly. But first I want to address a different kind of "booster"—one your immune system needs sometimes to make vaccines more efficient: adjuvants.

DR. BOB SAYS

Like booster seats in a car, booster shots are designed to enhance your safety. They are based on science and learning and are not evidence of any mistake or flaw in vaccines. Miss your booster shot, and you are inadequately protected and run a risk of getting an infection, albeit a weaker one.

WHAT ARE ADJUVANTS? AREN'T THEY DANGEROUS?

One of the nice things about the mRNA COVID-19 vaccines is that they work perfectly on their own. They did not need *adjuvants,* or the addition of substances like aluminum salt (the most common vaccine adjuvant and used for nearly a century) to boost the immune system response and make the vaccine more efficient. When the antigen or organism used in a vaccine fails to produce a huge immune response on its own and the antibodies disappear quickly, adjuvants prevent that, probably by acting on those dendritic cells. Aluminum is such a good adjuvant that it also stimulates the immune response to whooping cough and diphtheria, which is why they are often given together in the Tdap vaccine.

The body has some natural adjuvants or immune boosters, too, like the biomes or the microbial organisms of the bowel and gut we covered in Chapter 2, which research has shown is extremely important to vaccine efficacy. For example, when investigators noted that children from poorer countries or low socioeconomic groups did not respond well to the trivalent flu vaccine in contrast to children from wealthier countries and upper-income groups, the quality of intestinal microbiota was thought to be directly involved. Early data also showed that the efficacy of vaccines was less in germ-free mice and mice treated with antibiotics, conditions which would destroy the natural microbial population of the bowel. Studies of genetically identical twins show that they have different immune responses to a vaccine, which most likely depended on those microbial populations or environmental factors, and not their genetics as previously thought. All this reemphasizes the importance of a healthy gut, but these and other natural adjuvants are not enough of a boost. So, we turn to additives.

The use of adjuvants is not without controversy, however, thanks in part to some insinuation around the pertussis vaccine in the 1970s and other associations. There are also allegations that multiple immunizations and the presence of added adjuvants result in a wide variety of chronic systemic autoimmune diseases. In the end, there is little, if any, evidence to support a connection to any of these or other insinuated adjuvant side effects.

My friend and colleague Arthur Brawer discusses these unfortunate associations very clearly in his 2019 paper, "Hidden Vaccine Toxicity." Aside from aluminum, he notes that 20-plus vaccines contain *polysorbate-80* (sodium dihydrogen phosphate dihydrate) and other *immunostimulatory compounds* or ISCOMs. All these compounds contain organo-siloxanes, a form of silica or silicon dioxide, which you might recall from silicone breast implants are alleged to be adjuvants for the immune system and suspected as causes of other immune diseases like scleroderma, rheumatoid arthritis, lupus, and other lesser-known conditions.[3] When it comes to vaccines, the concern was that organo-siloxanes can produce a residuum of something called sorbitol, a sugar often found in fruits and vegetables. While this compound *can* produce significant side effects when given to excess, vaccines are not vehicles for anything close to the significant amount of sorbitol needed to produce those effects.

---

[3] Data produced from women with silicone breast implants resulted in concerns regarding inserts, and women were asked to have them removed and replaced every 10 to 15 years. Their association with diseases of immunity were never confirmed. Anecdotal reports are common, and I have seen suggestions in my own involvement with patients.

> ### DR. BOB SAYS
>
> Don't hang your concerns about vaccines on adjuvants. They are very necessary to allow your immune system to get that vaccine "spark of joy" that will protect you. The science around their side effects is limited and often dubious.

THERE *ARE* SIDE EFFECTS TO VACCINES—ISN'T THAT BAD?

As I have and will say throughout this book, there are trade-offs to any medications and treatments and vaccines are no exception: There *are* side effects and always will be, and they are totally understandable and expected to some degree in everyone like the sore arm at the site of the injection many of us experience. In the COVID-19 vaccinations, most side effects ran from rashes to muscle and joint pain to a feverish, sleepless night. As with most side effects, those were, by and large, short-lived and relieved with acetaminophen, aspirin, or antihistamines. While some people have severe allergic reactions to vaccines, just as they do to eggs or shellfish, many of these can be avoided or are instantly recognized and treated.

But here's the most important thing to know about those and all those vaccine side effects: *They are good. They are signs of your immune system working.*

Yes, even those rare blood clots that temporarily halted the use of the Johnson & Johnson vaccine in the United States and caused panic over the AstraZeneca vaccine in Europe are now explained. Those clots commanded headlines worldwide, and they were bad. But they were also the immune system in action. Though the reason or reasons for these abrupt reactions are unclear, we should herald them as proof that the biological soul is working—alerting you to danger and providing information to doctors that could save you and others.

Let's break down that side effect that caused so much concern in 2021: vaccine-induced immune thrombotic thrombocytopenia or the loss of platelets and the formation of small clots in the veins of the brain a week to two weeks after receiving the Johnson & Johnson vaccine. Platelets have a substance on their surface called platelet factor 4, and this appears to be the "antigen" that the Johnson & Johnson vaccine patients who experienced the severe side effect saw as foreign. (We do see this antiplatelet factor 4 randomly in patients treated with regular molecular weight heparin, the most common blood thinning medication, which is why you might have heard stories of doctors being asked not to treat patients that might be suffering from this vaccine reaction with heparin.) The reaction is exceedingly rare.

Another reversible reaction to the viral vector vaccine from Johnson & Johnson is the exceptionally rare Guillain Barre Syndrome or transient immune attack on peripheral nerves with resulting paralysis.

Platelets, or *thrombocytes*, are particles that come from cells called *megakaryocytes* that help blood clot. If they fall to extremely low levels, it can lead to bleeding that won't stop and can be serious even with a simple nosebleed or a cut when shaving. The *thrombocytopenia* at the heart of vaccine-induced immune thrombotic thrombocytopenia means a low blood platelet count, which is rare in adults and a common aspect of many autoimmune diseases. The autoimmune form of *thrombocytopenia* is called *immune thrombocytopenic purpura* or ITP, which affects kids and adults, and most parents know is something that requires the assistance of a pediatrician.

As adults, the autoimmune reaction can lead to serious uncontrolled bleeding but even that is exceedingly rare. That's why these low platelet levels and clots were not caught in the second and third phases of trials: They are, and continue to be, exceedingly rare. Of the first 6.7 million doses of the Johnson & Johnson vaccine given in the United States, *six* people, all women, developed blood clots in the venous sinus of the brain, which works out to fewer than one in a million. Four of the women affected were treated and released, one ended up in critical condition, and one died. By contrast, according to *Science Translational Medicine*

(2020), more than 50 percent of all infected patients clot off parts of their lungs after a COVID-19 infection.

Of course, it is completely fair to ask: How can that blood clot in the brain or anywhere else if there are no platelets to help it clot? The answer is there are other antibodies or triggers that concurrently produce clots. That's why I suggested that every patient with COVID-19 take aspirin from the outset of their symptoms to prevent clotting. If you take aspirin (even baby aspirin), you chemically affect the platelets and prevent clotting in small and perhaps even large vessels.[4] I have also suggested that all nonvaccinated COVID-19 patients admitted to the hospital have their blood thinned with low-dose heparin or another novel blood thinner because the clotting issue in the small vessels of the lung is a major reason for severe complications, disabilities, and fatalities. Another significant but rare reaction to vaccines happens in young men (mostly below the age of 18): inflammation of the heart muscle (myocarditis) or the lining of the heart (pericarditis). This is undoubtably related to an activated immune system and perhaps some autoimmunity, as pericarditis and myocarditis are among the most common cardiac events in patients with autoimmunity.

I could go on, but it would take dozens, if not hundreds, of pages to similarly break down all the reactions from the common to the rare, the minor to the major from vaccines—and to dismiss all the bogus claims. (Heard the one about neurological pain and fatiguing syndromes being linked to vaccines? No data exists to support this.) I could explain once again that trade-offs are inevitable with any medication and then get addressed like with the pertussis vaccine, which did affect tens of thousands of children. I could go through some of the debacles of decades or more than a century ago like mutations causing vaccine viruses to revert to being infectious and cause disease or vaccines containing

---

[4] Many doctors advise their patients under 70 to include an 81mg baby aspirin in with their daily vitamins and other medications to prevent stroke and heart attacks unless they are at risk for increased bleeding.

a not-so-weak virus causing the disease, which is what happened in a very few cases with Albert Sabin's oral polio vaccine. Much of this insinuation is just people looking for an answer as to why vaccines are bad, not why they are good.

In some ways, I get it. Reactions can be unpredictable, and uncertainty, no matter how rare, is hard and uncomfortable, but it should not be taken as evidence that vaccines are dangerous. Vaccines affect the immune system in marvelous ways and depend on many things within the human body to facilitate their actions.

If I were a betting man, I would say the revving up of the immune system is not surprising but caused by the MHC class I T cells and likely the natural killer T cells we discussed previously, which are different in everybody and one of the reasons reactions vary from person to person: The immune system behaves differently in different people under different conditions, which I chalk up to something called immunogenetics or the heredity of the immune system (which I cover in the next chapter). But there are other factors like parasitic infections, diarrheal diseases, and even malnutrition that lower the overall efficacy of a vaccine. The indiscriminate use of antibiotics in some cultures in infants can have a major effect on their inability to withstand infections after immunization (and another reason why antibiotics should not be used indiscriminately).

Our inability to predict who might be severely affected by a vaccine is the same inability to predict who might die from certain bacterial or viral infections because of the unique nature of each soul, both spiritual and biological. But when we connect the dots between patients who have similar genetic or other markers, we can at least prepare for the worst. Of course, the preparation for any ill effects from vaccines starts during the planning for a vaccine and considers such major factors as age (with infants and young children and the elderly getting special consideration because of the state of their immune systems) and pregnancy. A pregnant woman's immune system defends her and her baby from infection, and immunity is passed from mother to baby in the form of antibodies. The vaccines that should *not* be given to pregnant mothers include those for HPV or human papilloma virus, MMR or measles, mumps, and rubella, and varicella. It is perfectly safe, however, for and all expecting mothers should get a flu vaccine and a Tdap vaccine (in the third trimester) to protect the baby from whooping cough.

COVID-19 vaccines were not approved for children under the age of 16 in the initial emergency use but started to be soon after, and we now know are safe for pregnant mothers, especially those at special risk for serious infection. Clinical trials with infants, toddlers, and young children for COVID-19 vaccines lagged behind those for adults because, in the reverse of most viral infections, children were less susceptible and often asymptomatic. But it is still important to vaccinate them when the time comes and not just to protect them from transmitting the disease to others or the virus adapting and changing its victim profile in the future. For example, some children get multisystem inflammatory syndrome (MIS-C) that is thought to be an overreaction to the virus by the immune systems, another demonstration that the biological soul is never the same in anyone.

As for the elderly and those with comorbid conditions, that is a no-brainer for vaccines like those for COVID-19. The elderly need vaccination as a way of preventing death as they inevitably experience immune system senescence (though people with extreme senescence might not respond to vaccines). Those with comorbid conditions like chronic obstructive lung disease, congestive heart failure, or malignant conditions like leukemia or lymphoma, must be protected against severe infection with any organism, but particularly viruses like COVID-19, which prefers to attack the lungs but does not spare the kidneys or hearts and even the brains of those infected.

Doctors and researchers are also prepared to understand a host of factors that you may or may not be aware of when it comes to vaccines. For example, the nasal "live" flu vaccine should never be given to anyone on anticancer drugs or other immunosuppressive medicine that prevent B cells or T cells from working effectively. People with not enough T or B cells due to medicines have a 55 percent chance of death from any endemic virus like the flu, COVID-19, or measles. Patients on B cell inhibitors like Rituxan or anticancer drugs like Gazyva or Imbruvica also should not get live vaccines. Their immune systems have no way to respond to the virus being injected, and consequently, it could produce a serious infection.[5]

If all this is not enough, passive surveillance programs are in place to monitor vaccine safety and effectiveness and the reporting of family members, manufacturers, and health care facilities and providers. As you might expect, people looking for a reason to distrust vaccines will argue that this passive surveillance is unreliable and inaccurate, arguing that chronic diseases occur months and years after immunization and that the data are flawed. But what's flawed is the negative approach they take. Even the most extreme reactions to vaccines are a sign of the biological soul working. I believe the immune system gets so revved up by the administration of the vaccine in some people that the body begins to have this autoimmune phenomenon.

I feel for every life lost, but every sacrifice has an altruistic silver lining: now that we know what to look for, we can be ready when it happens again. Yet vaccine skeptics and, honestly, the media looking to get ahead of a story, jump on this as *the* reason not to be vaccinated. That ignores that every day you (or your children) and many others have a much bigger risk of dying or getting seriously hurt by other choices you make—getting behind the wheel of a car (and especially not wearing a seatbelt), texting while driving or even walking, swimming with no lifeguard or supervision—and you don't have doctors and nurses watching you or on call if something bad happens.

---

[5] If you or someone you know is on a drug or biological that inhibits their immune response, you could get a monoclonal antibody against the spike protein or convalescent plasma, which could protect you from the acute symptoms of COVID-19 and other pathogens. Regeneron, producers of the original monoclonal antibody, was effective at decreasing symptomatic infections of COVID-19, but it did not work for every single person. People with combined immunodeficiency, a condition where antibodies are not made to anything in large amounts, should contact their doctors as well.

I am not saying COVID-19 vaccines are perfect—no vaccines are. But they are highly effective and, like almost all vaccines throughout history, have been better than the alternative. While there were COVID-19 "breakthrough" infections, they are thankfully rare: According to the Centers for Disease Control, only 5,800 of the first 75 million Americans fully vaccinated against COVID-19 contracted the virus, and the odds of dying went almost to zero. Like all new medications or procedures, there were downsides to the vaccines. Some of the side effects like those blood clots or the heart inflammation *sounded* devastating, but I heard anecdotally that you were far more likely to be in a serious car accident driving to get a vaccine than get a side effect from the vaccine itself.

DR. BOB SAYS

Every drug or biological you take has a trade-off. Vaccines can and do have side effects, usually very minor. Realize these side effects are your immune system recognizing the vaccine's presence. Depending on your genetics, you will respond extremely well or moderately well to your vaccination. Either way, death and serious illness are rare after vaccination and most side effects are MUCH more preferable to the infection itself.

WHY DO WE STILL FEAR VACCINES?

As you probably heard countless times, the goal in coming out of the COVID-19 pandemic and ending a seemingly endless series of lockdowns and restrictive protocols is herd immunity. Herd immunity can be achieved in two ways: that percentage of the population can be infected, leading to unacceptable deaths (as was the case with the Spanish flu); or that percentage of people get vaccinated so that the virus has fewer people to infect, and the chain of transmission is broken.

Remember: A virus needs a live body to keep growing. The only way to stop it is death or lowering the number of susceptible members of a population and preventing those who are not vaccinated from being infected. I have preferred the latter since I was a child and had my summers taken away by polio. I can still hear my mother making me avoid swimming holes. Polio was finally obliterated by Jonas Salk's injectable vaccine and Sabin's oral version. The vaccines led to herd immunity from the horrible paralysis occurring randomly in young children and eventually polio was eradicated in the United States. And we were grateful. There was nothing dramatically polarizing about it. That is untrue about almost everything today.

How polarizing has the idea of some vaccinations become? Let me say this: I give equal credit to President Trump's Operation Warp Speed for the development of the emergency-use COVID-19 vaccines and President Biden for the focus and messaging around the rollout that had every American age 12 and over eligible for a vaccine by the middle of 2021. That I credited both administrations probably alienated readers on both sides. That I would like to see both presidents sit together and congratulate one another for their roles but that seems like a pipe dream.

Whether we like it or not, our politics are highly partisan, but COVID-19 and every other virus, parasite, and bacteria that infect our bodies are not partisan. I'm not saying that either administration's efforts were perfect, but neither were the COVID-19 vaccines approved for emergency use. But they were highly effective. Yet still we fear vaccines, and it is a fear I know well beyond COVID-19.

I have been the volunteer emergency director of my local ambulance corps for years, and as such, I have been tasked with giving our fire and police departments their yearly flu vaccine. Our bravest and finest line up every year, and I can see the fear on their faces and the questions behind their eyes: *What about the aftereffects? Will I get the flu? Why should I risk taking something that might not even stop me from getting the flu?* Some refuse to be inoculated, even though their jobs demand that they interact with people who could be infected. In COVID-19, the resistance, at least initially, was even stronger: *I do not want to be the first. I do not want to be the guinea pig. I don't trust the government. Do I take a vaccine, for which I have significant reservations, or suffer the possible consequences of getting a disease that will kill me at the worst and possibly make me critically ill for many months and I can still get infected?*

Again, I get it. These were (and still are) the words of many people in the uncertainty of the COVID-19 pandemic. I could provide them with a litany of scientific information: the research done and the participants in studies; details on the mostly mild side effects; and the need to achieve herd immunity necessary to truly lift pandemic restrictions and protect themselves and their families. Maybe I get the ones who resist to sign up for a shot with, "Okay, it's better than dying of this terrible disease." That's a start. Maybe they then tell others in their community who are hesitant to do the same.

Even with the vaccines we have now, the future is not "safe." Viruses never disappear. They can evolve. They can jump species. There are many diseases for which no vaccine exists like TB, malaria, HIV, and schistosomiasis (a parasitic infestation common to developing countries). Even pathogens like smallpox might never go away and could make a comeback with a few adjustments. Polio has. It was on the verge of being eradicated in 2015 and now rogue variants to the vaccine-derived strains are turning up around the world. But unlike the eighteenth and early nineteenth centuries, we now have deep understanding and technology to adjust these vaccines to continue to protect us from infection. Unless they put your health at risk or you truly have a profound religious objection, get them.

Genetics and Immunity
Self from Nonself

Why do viral infections and diseases kill some people and not others? Why is there so much variation in the outcome of infections? Why do some people and, in many cases, whole families suffer disastrous consequences from infections and others mild or even no symptoms? I lost count long ago how many times I was asked these questions during the recent global pandemic. The answer is complicated and not just for COVID-19, but also for influenza, measles, and other infections. Several factors covered elsewhere in this book play a part, such as age (older people were devastated by COVID-19 while young people were largely unaffected like they are by the flu), the health and state of your immune system including the presence of any comorbidities (another disease or condition like diabetes or cancer), and environmental influences (smoking and ingestion of alcohol and drugs, both illicit and medical). But I suspect that this variation in our immune systems is also driven by your genetics—the barcodes of life inherited from members of your family the moment sperm meets egg that make every biological soul unique.

Genetics is at the heart of the immune system. It is the plan, the guidebook, the architectural masterpiece that makes you who you are and, among other things, directs your immune system as if you had a GPS implanted inside you. Your genetics direct how you handle infections, inflammation, the response to diseases and their integration as you age, and the overall quality and length of your life. We can now understand why certain people succumb to certain infections and not others by studying these genetics.

I'll consider two kinds of genetic effects on immunity in this chapter:

- The genetics you inherit from your biological family, like skin color or eye color. What Charles Darwin called "regular inheritance." These genetics are a permanent part of your being.
- Epigenetics, or genetics influenced by behavior and environment. What I call "temporary inheritance" or heredity of the moment.

Everyone has the potential to inherit disease through regular inheritance, whether because of "glitches" in your immune function, inherited proteins, or missing genes. Epigenetics refers to the altered expression of your genes in cells outside of, and even despite, regular inheritance. With regular inheritance, your DNA can change over time; in temporary inheritance, the *expression* of your DNA changes—you have the same genes, but each reacts differently as a result of a subtle alteration of materials surrounding the genes.

Epigenetics (or "imprinting" as it was once called) is a recent concept and a powerful way to understand how genes can alter immune function. I've used it throughout this book when talking about stress, living conditions, diet, and the medicines you ingest, all of which can have epigenetic effects. What we have learned with epigenetics and genetics overall is revolutionary when it comes to the intricacies of your immune system's response to insults and organisms, maintaining recognition of self from nonself, and what it does when confronted with unknown infections. It is also a bit scary because it gives us the grand design of our future and past and predicts the future of our offspring when it comes to inherited disease. Understanding what all of this means for our biological soul—and the possibilities for changing these regular and temporary genetic expressions—begins with a short understanding of genetics itself.

There are two kinds of genetics: regular and temporary. Your regular genetics comes from adaptation over time and is called Darwinian genetics. It's permanent. Your temporary genetics is called epigenetics, which means your genes are altered by events or substances over a defined period of time, not forever.

GENETICS: REGULAR INHERITANCE

Genetics is the study of genes, those definitive collections of nucleic acids orderly arrayed on chromosomes that sit in each of your cells. It is a relatively recent science. Heredity or biological inheritance, the passing of physical and mental traits from one generation to another, has been understood for thousands of years. But the understanding of genes and biological individuality only started in the nineteenth century, crystallized during the early twentieth century, and exploded exponentially from there with vast growth in the knowledge of basic molecular biology.

The concept of evolutionary biology belongs to Charles Darwin and *On the Origin of Species* (1859), but Gregor Mendel is considered the founder of modern genetics and the concept of inheritance of simple traits. An Augustinian friar and abbot in a small monastery in Brno, Moravia (part of the Czech Republic today), Mendel loved to garden and, while growing pea plants for the refectory's dinners, became interested in their horticultural variations. His experiments from 1856 to 1863 went well beyond the crossbreeding farmers had been doing with plants and animals. Focusing on seven specific characteristics including pod and seed shape and color, he noticed that traits like pea and leaf color were passed on from parent pea plants to their offspring.

Mendel's rules of heredity—the laws of Mendelian inheritance describing the passing of genetic traits from one living thing to another—percolated for decades through the work of many scientists, who eventually coined the terms gene and genetics in the early twentieth century. That's when Thomas Hunt Morgan, an American evolutionary biologist and geneticist building on the Mendelian laws of inheritance through the study of fruit flies, identified and named the *chromosome,* the carrier of hereditary characteristics and the link between genes (for which he received the Nobel Prize in Physiology or Medicine in 1933). Morgan's work described the role of sex chromosomes that determine whether you are biologically male (an X and Y chromosome) or female (XX chromosome). But it took many more years and scientists to identify the hereditary package of 46 chromosomes that every human cell has a within its nucleus, only two of which are related to your sex. The other 44 are called constitutive or nonsex chromosomes, 22 of which are inherited equally from father and mother.

All these chromosomes are composed of *deoxyribonucleic acid,* or DNA, the molecule which consists of chains that coil around each other to form the double helix familiar to most of us today. Discovered in the 1950s by James Watson and Francis Crick, DNA is your personal barcode, specifically arranged on a skeleton of sugars (*deoxyribose*). It has four nucleotide bases (guanine, cytosine, thymidine, and adenine) that give everyone's genes endless combinations. Acquired from your parents, grandparents, and great-grandparents, your DNA carries your unique biological instructions.[1] Fixed and compacted as though carved in stone in your cells, it is the substance of which your genes are made and never

---

[1] I had two brushes with genetic history. When I was at Roosevelt Hospital, the office down the hall belonged to a kindly old man named Erwin Chargaff, who was retiring and welcomed one of my postdoctoral fellows moving into his office. Only later did I understand that Chargaff realized that DNA was the substance of the gene and discovered that the proportions of bases in DNA varied with the species from which they came, seminal work that later allowed Watson and Crick to discover the double helix. My other brush with genetic history involved my friend Maclyn McCarty, a professor at Rockefeller University who, together with Oswald Avery and Colin MacLeod, discovered the "transforming principle." This principle showed that DNA was transformative in bacteria and that genes could be moved from one bacterium to another, transferring hereditary characteristics with it.

changes as you live and age. Whether you are pope or peasant, your genes are influenced by other genes and DNA sequences (and sometimes linked together), but they are immutable on the inside.

In genetic and now molecular biology dogma, DNA transcribes ribonucleic acid or RNA, which then acts as DNA's protein messenger, specifying the sequence of protein synthesis via a mini machine called a ribosome. This is DNA expression. However, in some viruses, RNA, not DNA carries the genetic information, which is why in the COVID-19 global pandemic we heard so much about "messenger RNA" or mRNA vaccines. The injection of these mRNA vaccines was nothing short of a revolution that depended on our clear knowledge of how chromosome 6 and the immune system work. So, how does it work?

DR. BOB SAYS

Regular genetics is the way that we inherit our family traits like hair, skin, and eye color, as well as genetically based diseases like muscular dystrophy.

GENETICS AND IMMUNITY: MOLECULAR MARVELS

While immunology and genetics both began to be studied in the nineteenth century, immunogenetics—the study of the genetic basis of immune response—started in the 1970s and took off in the twenty-first century. As a result, many of the molecular events surrounding the presentation of antigens and the genetic connection to autoimmune diseases are just coming to light. But already those connections are significant and might be some of, if not *the* most, important aspects of being immunity strong in the future.

Most of the immune response genes are located on chromosome 6, one of the biggest and most active parts of the human genome.

It contains some 200 genes, each with 4×10^6 base pairs in the immune site. Antiviral proteins like interferons and complement components that amplify or "complement" an immune reaction (and the recognition of self and nonself) all begin with the DNA on chromosome 6. These genes are polymorphic, meaning that there are seemingly endless unique copies of these genes and no two people are alike. In fact, among genes, these are possibly the most varied of any other part of the genome in the body. The location of these immune response genes on chromosome 6 includes the *major histocompatibility complex*, or MHC.[2]

Your MHC rules your immune system. Its genes and the molecules they produce or encode are what give your immune system individuality and tell you not only of your compatibility with another person but also what is self and nonself and what invaders are good or bad. Because MHC genes are polymorphic and given the enormous number of genes and base pairs programmed into you, no one—not even from the same family—has identical immune response genes to others in the family. But regular inheritance explains why your uncle by blood is much more likely than your aunt by marriage to be able to donate a kidney to you. Your uncle has inherited many or most of the immune response genes that you have, and his immune system sees you as "compatible."[3]

---

[2] Chromosome 6 includes many other genes that may or may not have relevance to immunity, but the most important genes are related to the MHC. The prefix *histo* means "tissue"; the MHC was discovered during tissue transplantation experiments.

[3] The MHC is part of the human leukocyte antigen (HLA) or white blood cell antigen network discovered early in immunology through antigenic differences between white blood cells. Everything on the HLA is categorized by letters: HLA A, B, C, D . . . followed by a number. HLA B27 individuals have an interesting bone condition called *ankylosing spondylitis* or reactive arthritis. This gene on chromosome 6 tells the immune system to react to bacterial antigens in a certain way to cause tendonitis and back pain. This gene locus on the chromosome reacts with a peptide from a foreign organism (usually a bacterium like salmonella or yersinia). The foreign protein binds to the MHC and is processed as a foreign antigen, which in the presence of this HLA gene, results in chronic crippling pain and stiffness. One year, a water station at the New York Marathon was contaminated with *yersinia enterocolitica*, which was discovered only after investigation by the New York City Health Department after several runners came down with reactive arthritis. Thankfully, only the few runners who carried MHC HLA B27 and drank the water came down with the diseases because of their immunogenetics.

Your genes control the show. Whether you are compatible with members of your family or have some unfortunate glitches that allow you to have an inherited disease depends on your genes which are on chromosomes. As far as your biological soul is concerned, chromosome 6 is where the action is.

The MHC genes on chromosome 6 are referred to as MHC class I or MHC class II and are among the most varied series of genes on the entire chromosome. MHC class I genes are found on all your cells and are most important for presentation of foreign materials (viruses like the flu or COVID-19 or antigens like a bacterial cell) to a specific T cell population (usually cells with a CD8 marker on them). The T cells then show them to the rest of the immune system, alerting your natural killer T cells that another cell has changed for the worse, meaning it has been infected by a virus or even changed to a cancer cell and must be eliminated. MHC class II genes are found on B cells, macrophages, and dendritic cells and are probably the most important genes for transplantation of tissues. These molecules present the foreign invaders to helper T cells (those that have a CD4 marker on them) for them to determine what to do with it.

We can now determine the location and character of these MHC loci through molecular testing. In the old days, we determined immune compatibility with sera in a Terasaki plate (named after Paul Terasaki, a pioneer in organ transplantation at UCLA). These plates allowed the rapid determination of tissue compatibility, using small amounts of sera that told us whether an organ donor was compatible with a recipient. With molecular testing, life became much easier for most transplant laboratories. We no longer had to ship sera from multiparous women from countries around the world to identify their MHC molecules and use their blood as reagents in the lab to find out if people were compatible (usually women with more than eight children who made their own antibodies to MHCs of their children during pregnancy). With knowledge of DNA and RNA, doctors like me can do the typing in a small dish and can see your MHC molecules in gels that I create and stain.

When it comes to diseases, your genes code for antibodies or immunoglobulins, which have specific structures in each of us that are directed to foreign substances. Again, MHC genes are polymorphic and vary from person to person, meaning that we all have endless varieties of MHC molecules that bind to proteins in attempts to regulate immunity. These genes also code for the lymphocyte receptors that are critical to your immune system's innate and adaptive response responsible for recognizing self from nonself, combating viral infections, regulating inflammation, and giving orders to dendritic cells or antigen-presenting cells as to who is friend or foe. Foreign peptides encounter the specific MHC on lymphocytes and instructions are transmitted to other cells and tissues that there is a potential criminal to confront.

All I just covered is a massive simplification of the MHC complexity but hits at the most important part for immunogenetics: MHC affects all antigenic recognition, immune surveillance, and our ability to fight most invaders.

Consider also immunogenetics when it comes to what we learned about vaccine research and protection against viruses and the questions that started this chapter. The true danger of the COVID-19 infection was—and remains—the unpredictable effects of the infection on certain people and why this can vary from individual to individual and family to family. Entire families have been destroyed by COVID-19, while others are asymptomatic and even immune. I am particularly dumbfounded by the deaths of otherwise healthy young men and women who have no comorbidities and succumb to this disease, which is why I side with the considerable speculation that these deaths are due to immunogenetic glitches that are not apparent until the infection occurs.

My colleagues at Rockefeller have started research on something called IEI, or inborn errors of immunity, which could explain some of these abnormal responses to a simple viral invasion. Some examples might be the genetics of interferon (an antiviral cytokine) or the nuances of cellular recognition (based on regular genetics inherited from someone who succumbed to the pandemic of 1918). Such immune responses might be substantially different in young or old people, or even entire families. In other cases, people of all ages may lack the ability to make a neutralizing antibody or have an MHC that is defective because of a missing protein on the receptor that prevents their cells from communicating. As if to emphasize my point, I wrote that sentence the day a 97-year-old woman infected with COVID-19 walked out of my hospital, while a healthy 22-year-old tennis pro came in with respiratory failure from the virus and died. These stark contrasts in our immune responses make indelible clinical impressions.

Perhaps the most striking example of a regular genetic disturbance—and one population that is most vulnerable to COVID-19 infection, which I rarely get asked to talk about—shows that some genes outside of chromosome 6 are important to immunity: people with Down syndrome. Those with this genetic disorder have three copies of chromosome 21 (called trisomy 21)—three copies of a gene that allows COVID-19 easy entry into your cells. Natural killer T cells do not develop properly in the biological soul of people with Down syndrome and the number of circulating B cells (the sources of antibody through the plasma cells they become) is exceptionally low. As a result, those with Down syndrome live in a state of chronic inflammation and can easily succumb to infection by COVID-19.

At least now, thanks to our knowledge of RNA, we not only created remarkably effective vaccines for emergency use quicker than anyone thought possible, but also had polymerase chain reaction or PCR testing, which was created in 1985 and became essential and virtually common knowledge during the COVID-19 pandemic. PCR tests are incredibly accurate at determining viral infection by detecting RNA specific to a virus—within days at first and then hours of infection—whether or not a person has any symptoms. In PCR tests, a single set of viral genes is amplified using molecular means to give a simple answer of infected or not. This would be unthinkable to me when I started my medical career.

Simply put, the inner workings of the biological soul are being dissected and redefined every decade, leading to the biggest questions of all: *Can it be changed? Can we remove the glitches in our genes that leave us vulnerable to COVID-19 and any foreign invader?* The answer is, for the most part, yes. The next question is: How far do we want to go?

A BIOLOGICAL MOONSHOT: THE SLICING AND DICING OF GENES

What I said before about the biological dogma of your genetics applies from the inside out, but the rise of molecular genetics has allowed scientists to tinker with genetics from the outside in. This manipulation became feasible at the end of the twentieth century and today allows us to cut and paste genes in individual cells like we would text in a word processing document. One of the most relevant to immunology and medicine was the advent of recombinant DNA technology, the technology for which was invented in the 1970s and subsequently allowed scientists to make certain drugs that act within the body to control immune function.

Today, we can splice together selected genes, just like you would the end of two wires, and create customized chromosomes. We can even enter cells and perhaps change the nature of heredity. The 2020 Nobel Prize in Chemistry was awarded to Emmanuelle Charpentier and Jennifer A. Doudna, who discovered and developed the CRISPR technology. CRISPR stands for clustered regularly interspaced short palindromic repeats, which is basically longhand for molecular or genetic "scissors" that the Nobel committee rightly noted could be the sharpest tool yet for "rewriting the code of life."

CRISPR technology allows us to cut and paste *within* a genome with ease, allowing genetic repair of glitches—the broken or defective genes within all areas of the body, but particularly within the immune system. The technology is based on a bacteria's way of protecting itself. Bacteria have their own immune protection against viruses that invade them called *bacteriophage*. Charpentier and Doudna explored bacteria's ability to make this genetic barrier to an invading virus and then cut that virus to pieces with a protein enzyme called Cas-9. CRISPR then uses the bacterial technique of matching nucleic acid (RNA with DNA) strands to specific invasive phage genes and then clips the unwanted strands and replaces them with preferred designed gene clusters. In other words, they use the bacteria's way of protecting itself from the inside out to slice and dice genes from mammalian cells from the outside in.

The first CRISPR experiments on human embryos occurred in 2015. A few clinical trials on treating cancer and blood disorders started in 2019. There are also experiments being done in which CRISPR changes genes *within* the body, not by removal and replacement. All the research points to incredible possibilities! But in spite of a global scandal surrounding a human trial in China in 2016, CRISPR has just the potential for altering regular genetics in each of our cells and offering a genetic cure for disease. Concern among ethicists involves changing the genomes of human embryos as they develop. We are far from that at the moment, but it is within reach.

The bigger question is, what does CRISPR mean for our evolution? James Watson said that our genetic instructions are simply the product of evolutions from times when we needed protection against certain infections that no longer exist, meaning our genomes were irrelevant in parts. I agree; we are a product of evolution. The potential for CRISPR to adjust our barcode of genetics going forward to have better control of disease is nothing short of a radical *revolution*, the culmination of decades of discussions of and research into biological engineering and surgically changing the genome by manipulating and changing genes. Before CRISPR, the results of genetic manipulation were of limited success and use (like providing proteins to hemophilia B patients to allow their blood to clot). CRISPR technology offered something different.

With CRISPR, it is now theoretically possible to change the MHC, the resistance to infections, the regular genetics inherited from your family, your production of cytokines, and even conditions like cancer. If we could cure AIDS by clipping the part of the gene that is affected by HIV, is that a good thing? I would say a firm yes as long as we focus on our greatest needs like curing disease and ethical, impeccable, transparent execution.

One thing is inarguable: the work on genetics and immunology has exploded because of molecular tools like CRISPR technology. But there is another field that focuses on the outside-in effect on genes and presents even more of a challenge: temporary inheritance.

EPIGENETICS: TEMPORARY INHERITANCE

When I say no person has the same antibody response to specific antigens, I mean it. It is even true for identical twins. Identical twins have chromosome 6 compatibility and can give their organs to one another without rejection. These identical genetics also lead to fun stories of them enjoying the same foods and the same personality traits of their mates, thinking alike, dressing alike, and feeling the same sensations, which for some of us can be quite "spooky." But their immune systems *are* different.

That identical twins have different immune responses and diseases allows for the idea that something other than regular heredity might be at play. Many diseases appear over time in one identical twin and not the other. These differences are likely the result of epigenetic change, meaning that their regular genetic elements, although identical, can be affected by modifications related to varied environments and behaviors after birth from what they eat to where they live to the medicines they take. Epigenetics is all about complexity and is a critical concept to explain the effects of the biome and the positive health benefits and negative effects diet, exercise, meditation, and stress on the immune system we covered in Chapter 2.

In fact, autoimmune diseases occur in both identical twins less than 50 percent of the time, suggesting other factors playing a role and over their lives. So, is the modification of the genes through epigenetic change the basis for these illnesses? If so, epigenetics represents a new frontier between the environment and the genome with regard to longevity.

But what exactly is epigenetics?

Epigenetics favors the idea that we adapt genetically to our environments and that certain traits can be acquired and passed on through one or several generations and then lost. Depending on your ethnicity (defined as the intrinsic elements of your heritage including your racial and/or cultural background), your family's exposure to infections decades ago could have influenced your genetic barcode for better or worse.

The idea of epigenetics dates to nearly half a century before Mendel planted his peas. Jean-Baptiste Lamarck proposed the idea that inheritance was not always the work of Darwinian adaptation and could be acquired and evolved from factors in the environment. For example, Darwin believed giraffes had long necks, because giraffes with long necks were genetically selected in favor of those with short necks. Lamarck did not believe that this natural selection was the law of evolution. He believed giraffes developed long necks because their environment required them to reach high into the eucalyptus trees to reach their leaves and eat. Moreover, he believed that these traits could be passed down to offspring.

Even at the time, Lamarck's ideas were quite controversial and remained so through the work of Mendel and Darwin, whose work gained favor over Lamarck. Genetics, after all, was immutable, right? Two centuries later, after the discoveries of recombinant DNA, the rise of molecular biology, and the chemistry of CRISPR, the controversy around Lamarckian inheritance disappeared, and his ideas became part of the foundation of epigenetics or heritable changes in the DNA expression in our genes—temporary expression that can go for one or more generations and then disappear. For example, it is likely that you will handle infections better because of your heritage. If your mother's family faced typhus in America during the nineteenth century, your genetic predisposition might be different from your friend whose great-grandfather had cholera in Britain or grandmother had TB in India. If your friend's ancestors overcame cholera in England in the late nineteenth century, then it is likely that they had a "natural" resistance, and this resistance could be passed on to your friend. In such cases, it is more likely to be epigenetics that is important to your fights against invaders than regular genetics.

The epi in epigenetics means above, which is directly connected to Lamarck's work. He believed all living things, not just giraffe necks, evolved in an upward direction. Lamarck, however, also believed that upward meant toward not just complexity, but perfection. We may not be chasing perfection when it comes to epigenetics today—one of the bigger concerns about CRISPR and what perfection even means—but epigenetics is changeable and something to produce health benefits or health defects as noted above if it can be used to change the pattern of regular genetic processes. In fact, CRISPR technology can also be applied to epigenetics, which may be just as important or more important to controlling disease. In *Nature* in 2016, Marianne Rots, a professor in Molecular Epigenetics at the University of Amsterdam in the Netherlands, who had been working on gene therapy and disease, explained why she started focusing on epigenetics: "I reasoned that many more diseases are due to disturbed gene expression profiles, not so much single gene mutations I had been focused on." In other words, adjusting the expression of genes would be more powerful than adjusting the genes themselves.

A well-known negative example of epigenetics was the famine that occurred in the Netherlands during World War II, when people starved due to Nazi blockades of food and coal. According to Siddhartha Mukherjee and his book *Gene*, the event came to be known as *hongerwinter* or the "hunger winter." Many died of malnourishment, but millions of people survived. Generations later, there were many health issues in the region like diabetes, obesity, and mental disease in the descendants of those survivors. As David Allis, a geneticist at Rockefeller University suggested, "Memory of metabolic stress could have become heritable," indicating that epigenetic change could affect populations as well as individuals.[4] Consider then today the scourge of malnutrition in poorer areas and underdeveloped countries or where the strife of war and tribal conflict is so common and not only a major cause of immunosuppression but likely has epigenetic effects on the immune system (as well as behavior) on future generations.

Simply put, our biological soul is impacted and affected, for better or worse, by our environment and behaviors and other lifestyle choices that are both a temporary modifier of our genes that have been inherited from generations of relatives and can be passed on to next generations. Dr. Michael Skinner, a professor at Washington State University, was among the first to show that chemicals could produce health effects across many generations without DNA changing. Using rats injected with substances that disturb endocrine hormones, he showed that fertility problems went along for multiple generations into grandchildren and then great-grandchildren and so on. He even suggested that epigenetic changes prepare children of future generations for the environment that they would be likely to encounter.

Science has said that sexual preference, creativity, and all of the changes one sees with altered immune function might in some way be modified by epigenetics. For example, sex hormones have epigenetic effects on us and may be the reason for the sex differences of the immune system and even the acquisition of disease. Or consider what scientists use to call epigenetics: "imprinting."

---

[4] A pioneer in this field was C. H. Waddington, a British developmental biologist who was fascinated by the differentiation of cells, namely why a *pluripotent cell* (capable of becoming anything in an embryo) simply decides to be a nerve cell instead of a skin cell or a cell in your retina and so on. He died before the concept of epigenetics was fully appreciated, but he was instrumental in giving oxygen to the theory called on to differentiate cells from pluripotent to those having specific roles might be operable here. In the laboratory we can change the direction of specialization based on some "force" that makes a retinal cell and a cell in your bowel different. I believe that this alteration of destiny of cells in a fetus in mom's womb can be affected by epigenetics, as you will see shortly.

Either the dad's or mother's genes are silenced during growth of the fetus, which is critical for normal development. A woman has two X chromosomes; one of them must be inactivated or silenced as part of a normal development. If it is not, as was discovered by Mary Lyon, a colleague of Waddington's, in 1961, immune aberrations can occur, which can result in autoimmune disease, which is one theory about why so many women have certain diseases when compared to men.

There are many ways in which these epigenetic changes might occur, and it comes down to subtle chemical changes that can have major effects on your DNA or on the chemicals called histones that allow the genes of DNA to wrap around it, affecting the DNA expression without altering its location or overall structure. Chemical modification of histones can result in altered expression of genes without substantially changing the DNA. The genes stay fixed and perfect, but the genetic expression of the gene changes. In chemical speak, these changes are methylation, acetylation, ubiquitylation, phosphorylation, and SUMOylation. Adding a chemical acetyl group or methylating proteins or carbamylating substances are all epigenetic ways to change expression of genes. Remember the dogma: DNA to mRNA to protein. The expression of the DNA to mRNA can be altered by subtle chemical changes of substances around and within the DNA, and though no genes are blinded or removed or cut out, the expression of them is altered and this can have profound effects on everything we do.[5]

There are many examples of these epigenetic changes in action, the most important of which is the effects of smoking. Cigarette smoking reduces DNA methylation levels at many loci on genes and the effect is reversible for some on cessation. If you ever asked about the mechanisms by which it was possible to prevent lung cancer by stopping smoking, this is it. In cancer, epigenetics has a major role to play by altering the genetic character of malignant

---

[5] Professor Moshe Szyf, a pharmacologist at McGill University, was the first to relate methylation of DNA to behavior, a concept he describes as "the adaptive mechanism of the genome."

cells through chemical means. With cigarette smoking, there are many changes because of tar in the smoke and enough chemical forced change in the body to produce altered cells and eventually tumors. Similar issues have come up with people eating barbecued foods. I don't want to ruin your summer barbecue, but the carbon produced by charring your hamburger has had some links to tumor-inducing activity because of metabolic studies of altered liver cell metabolism, so maybe cut back a little. Then there are the examples of Japanese people who eat a lot of smoked fish. They have disproportionate nasopharyngeal cancer due to the carbons in the fish. I could go on, but you get the point.

Alcohol abuse and the use of illicit drugs like heroin and cocaine have epigenetic effects on the immune system as well. Most drug users are immunosuppressed by definition and highly susceptible to deadly infections, but the effect is again reversible for some on cessation. Or maybe you don't drink or smoke or do drugs but are just feeling stressed? As I stated in Chapter 3, the effects of stress hormones on behavior are likely to be the most engaging epigenetic effects that humans relate to and why pursuits like yoga and meditation can chemically change the epigenetic effect of stress on the genome.

Finally, consider medications. We have seen throughout this book the impact that certain medications can have on the immune system and immune response, which the epigenetic response can alter. I published a paper 40 years ago on a drug called procainamide, which stabilizes the heart's rhythm and when given to certain people with slow liver metabolism developed a kind of reversible autoimmunity. As a rule, autoimmunity is *never* reversible, but a form of drug-induced lupus (widely known among physicians) is totally reversible because it was caused by a drug and cured by removing the drug. It seems that half of us are able by genetic mandate to remove the drug from our systems quickly, whereas the rest of us are very slow removing the drug. The people with slow metabolism did not chemically change the drug procainamide like the fast ones who attached an acetyl group to the drug.

This chemically induced autoimmunity was a simple illustration of epigenetic alteration of the immune response, producing disease in a few people via a chemical change.

I know this is a lot to process, but this is how epigenetics affects the immune system, immune diseases, and through immunity, cancer, heart disease, and possibly even dementia. T cells and the immune system continue to differentiate throughout life and into extremely old age. According to my colleague Dr. Bruce Richardson, a pioneering epigenetic immunologist, this depends on chemical reactions like DNA methylation or the adding of methyl groups to the DNA itself. This methylation is affected by many factors we have covered, such as stress and environmental factors like smoking, hunger, and infectious agents you encounter throughout your life. The natural killer T cell has *pluripotent capacity*, which means that it has a lot of potential. It can develop into one of several T cell lineages that can produce different cytokines like interferon against viruses or provide protection against cancer or certain parasitic infections, making their role crucial to keeping the immune system on track and preventing autoimmunity. All of these are regulated by epigenetic influences.

As it happens, the DNA in a cell is compressed by the sleeping bag of histones or proteins that allow the DNA to wrap around it called a nucleosome. The nucleosome cushions the DNA and allows or disallows gene expression. Many autoimmune diseases like Sjogren's syndrome, lupus, or multiple sclerosis include anti-histone antibodies, and drug-induced autoimmune diseases often show this antibody as a marker. The existence of these antibodies has never been explained, but I suspect the altered structure of the histone might become foreign to the immune system under certain circumstances. The genome can create identity, but the question before all of us is, *How?*

The Nobel laureate Walter Gilbert, a pioneering molecular biologist and leading proponent of the human genome project, is famous for opening his lectures by lifting a CD and telling his audience, "This is you." Gilbert was only half right. We are the data on that CD, but we are also everything that happens to us in the environment we live in and the choices we make. Everything you do, good or bad—from smoking and laying in the sun without sunscreen to eating right and exercise—has an effect on your genome and consequently your biological soul *and* the biological soul of your children and perhaps even those you influence either with stress or calm, just as your ancestors and others influenced yours. The MHC or the barometer that tells your immune cells how to handle bodily invaders, the genes that inform your T helper cells or natural killer cells, and the common identifier on each of your cells from neurons to lymphocytes are all identified and stored in your genome. They are ready to change and adapt to your environment. They influence your behavior and your longevity in ways we never imagined and that we are finally beginning to understand and accept.

DR. BOB SAYS

One of the most amazing aspects of epigenetics is its applicability to just about everything we know. Chemical or environmental alterations of gene expression can explain a great many alterations of behavior, disease expression, hormone effects, and even quirky mannerisms passed on in a couple of generations from relatives. Sit back and think about the changes that can evolve from your own environment. They are likely to be epigenetic.

9 Sex, Gender, Hormones, Pregnancy, and the Immune System

Let's talk politics! No, not Washington, D.C., but the politics of your body. The immune response of the biological sexes has many similarities, but their immune systems behave, well, like Democrats and Republicans. I know I said at the end of the vaccine chapter that infections are not partisan, but there is definitely a two-party system—man and woman—when it comes to the biological soul. What accounts for this dichotomy? Two factors: sex chromosomes and sex hormones, especially testosterone and estrogen. These hormones are exceedingly important to the development of the immune system, its properties during our adult lives, and the way we handle infections and other insults to our bodies like cancer and autoimmune disease.

The subject of sex always comes up when more women or men are affected by disease. It is why during the COVID-19 pandemic, both a trusted ear, nose, and throat doctor in Manhattan and the *New York Times* contacted me to talk about using estrogen to treat men facing end-of-life to prevent them from dying. Women, after all, far outlived men when faced with this severity of disease. Later, when the rare blood-clotting problems of the Johnson & Johnson and AstraZeneca COVID-19 vaccines skewed toward women and forced a halt to their distribution, I was constantly asked by the media, "Why mostly women?" Then, when the COVID-19 vaccine was given to young men and resulted in transient myocarditis and pericarditis, the question became, "Why young men?"

The story of COVID-19 and sex is just the most recent reason to me why there is no more interesting area within the immune diseases than the role of sex when it comes to immunity strong. In fact, it is of paramount importance and yet remains in many ways a puzzle with no solutions.

This chapter explores biological sex from several angles we have touched on in this book, including the role your biological sex plays in obtaining an autoimmune disease, immune resistance, and warding off diseases. It ends with a look at the marvel that is pregnancy and what it means for a woman's immune system. In between, this chapter also considers changes in gender using hormones. But please note I did not say that your gender is of paramount importance to immunity. For most of us, our biological sex controls much of what goes on during the day-to-day operation of our bodies and most importantly the immune system, and gender has little or nothing to do with it. Simply put, your sex is biology. Your gender is how you identify, appear to others, behave, and possibly your preference for sexual activity. That expression has no effect on your sexual biology. While injecting the hormones of the opposite sex and altering your sex-specific organs through surgery does impact your immune system, most people will never go through this, and even when they do, they will always be a man or a woman as far as their cells are concerned.

DR. BOB SAYS

Sex and gender are two different things and impact your immune system differently. But it is your biological sex that is unchangeable and is of paramount importance to disease expression.

YOUR BIOLOGICAL SEX AND DISEASE: 'TIS A PUZZLEMENT!

Here's the basic biology of sex: Women are born with a pair of X chromosomes, which we know from the last chapter are nucleic acids and proteins found in most living cells that carry our genetic information in the form of genes. Women are also usually born with an abundance of a *hormone* or chemical messenger called estrogen. Men are born with an X and a Y chromosome and usually an abundance of *androgens* or steroid hormones, the major one being testosterone. Most of us learned these facts in our first biology class. But we didn't need a book to see those hormones in action. They were expressing themselves all around us in the years-long process that is puberty.

Puberty is a time of hormonal fluctuations that start around 11 for most girls and 12 for boys. These fluctuations affect behavior and change your body's form well beyond pubic hair. Females grow breasts and start their periods as their ovaries, vagina, and uterus mature. Males become muscular, develop a lowered voice, start growing hair all over their body, and as any parent of a teenage boy knows, start stinking up every room in the home from their oily skin and sweat. All of this is basic stuff. What may not be obvious is that most autoimmune diseases begin at puberty and that women are at higher risk of getting these diseases right after puberty. What is not clear is how and why the emergence of these sex differences take on a new role in the immune system at the time of puberty. Sex hormones do have a role in making autoimmune and other diseases better or worse, promoting or inhibiting immune functions, but they cannot explain their causes. It is curious and confounding.

Henry G. Kunkel, my mentor and a renowned immunologist at Rockefeller University, was the first to clue me in to the role sex differences has on your immune system, including the fact that autoimmune diseases are more common to women than men. My own research on autoimmune diseases has shown this as well. For example, I have spent decades studying lupus (a disease that is very classically autoimmune and can destroy almost every system of the body), and there are no fewer than ten times as many women affected with the disease than men. There are many more of these diseases, many of which are not as widely known and some of which we touched on in this book including primary biliary cirrhosis (a terrible disease that attacks the liver), Sjogren's syndrome (in which the glands of the body are inflamed and the patient has little saliva or tears), and of course the most common autoimmune disease, rheumatoid arthritis (in which joints are destroyed and patients have to endure tremendous amounts of pain and immobility throughout their lives).

The question is: What role might hormones like estrogen play in these diseases? The answer eludes us, and some of the observations about what role sex differences play have been baffling.

A few years after the advent of the first oral contraceptive in the 1960s—which contained estrogen and progestin, a synthetic form of the progesterone hormone to prevent ovulation—physicians asked whether the advent of the "pill" had any major effects on rheumatoid arthritis manifestations. After all, it was found that some women who had rheumatoid arthritis tended to improve during certain times during menstruation when estrogens were the highest. In clinics, doctors would ask women about their symptoms and try to pair them with phases of their menstrual cycles. No surprise! Symptoms of rheumatoid arthritis like pain and fatigue were far worse right before the onset of the period. When the bleeding began, the symptoms abated. But in multiple clinical trials with women on and off oral contraceptives there was no measurable effect on the course of rheumatoid arthritis. And with lupus, many observations revealed the *reverse*: Symptoms would get worse right before the onset of the menstrual period and then improve with the onset of the period. In other words, symptoms varied by both disease state as well as from woman to woman.

The only consistency was that the vast majority of patients could predict exactly how they would feel when their periods would start and end based on their symptoms, which led me and many others to believe estrogen played a major role in modulation of disease activity. Estrogen levels also increase as a fetus grows in pregnancy, and plenty of evidence exists that women with rheumatoid arthritis (like Patricia at the start of this book) improve during pregnancy only to come crashing back as a vengeful disease after delivery when estrogen levels drop. Similarly, certain immune symptoms like rashes and Raynaud's syndrome disappeared during pregnancy, as estrogen does have anti-inflammatory effects.

These findings have made researchers look closely for more than a half-century at estrogen and women's immune function and to try and use estrogen to protect patients from rheumatoid arthritis and other diseases. There were plenty of misfires, like the use of birth control pills, which seemed to result in the decline of the incidence of rheumatoid arthritis. But causation was not correlation. Conversely, you might think that removal of female hormones would protect women from getting autoimmune disease. While that might be the case, it is a bit draconian to believe that every woman with an autoimmune disease should have a hysterectomy. But it is precisely what is done to certain animals that develop autoimmune disease. In fact, I was summoned by President George Herbert Walker Bush and First Lady Barbara Bush to see their springer spaniel, Millie. Millie had a litter of puppies, and after her pregnancy, developed lupus. I am not a veterinarian, but I do know lupus, so Dr. Burton Lee, the president's physician, asked what should be done for the First Dog of the United States. A veterinarian from the Bethesda Naval Hospital suggested Millie be spayed (have her ovaries removed). I concurred, and after the surgery, Millie not only recovered from her autoimmune disease with the help of a daily dose of cortisone, but also outlived her offspring.

That said, men succumb to infections before women, because women are able to fight viral infections with greater efficiency. Hence the suggestion of using estrogen to fight COVID-19. But would even a man near death consider having himself placed on female hormones or having his gonads removed to see another day? There is much more than biological politics in that decision. Yet, curiously, the idea of castration has problems when it comes to this idea. While chemical castration has been shown to lower sex drive in men, men who are infertile due to infection or traumatic removal of their gonads—thus lowering their testosterone—are actually *more* likely to acquire an immune disorder. Testosterone downregulates the immune system, so it is logical to assume that men who have had injury to their testes, the mumps, or a natural lack of androgens or male hormones could develop autoimmune symptoms such as joint pains and aches. This is indeed the case and data show that many men with autoimmune diseases have low levels of androgens due to injury, mumps, chronic alcoholism, or any other condition affecting their testicles that can lower the levels of male hormones in their bodies.

There have been experiments on men with autoimmune diseases, too, but they are rarer and no less satisfying in finding an absolute connection than those done on women. Some even connect to their chromosomes. Consider Klinefelter syndrome, a condition I have studied extensively that affects about 200,000 men worldwide. Men with Klinefelter syndrome have an extra copy of the X chromosome, making them XXY instead of XY.[1] A man who has this extra X chromosome has almost no female or male hormones and is 14 times more likely to acquire an autoimmune disease, which suggests that something about the X chromosome might have a role to play in autoimmune diseases, and not (just) hormones, and that hormones could point a way to a solution, if not a cure. However, sex chromosomes are sex-determining and use the same rules as other genes that influence a host of changes that depend upon them. The genes of chromosome 6, considered the immune response area of the genome, produce, and regulate the cells of the immune system, the production of antibodies, and

---

[1] Sadly, men with Klinefelter syndrome have no idea that they have it until they discover they cannot father children, gain weight in the wrong places, are passive aggressive, have erectile dysfunction at a young age, or develop an autoimmune disease prompting the doctor to take a good look at the patients' karyotype or chromosomes.

other important parameters of inflammation. It is also the site of a gene that regulates the metabolism of testosterone among other things.

There was once an idea that extra male hormones might help control the immune responses within patients with Klinefelter syndrome and autoimmunity. God knows I tried to do that with some of my patients, and all I succeeded in doing was increasing their atherosclerosis, making their necks and shoe sizes bigger, and triggering anger and aggression. One patient's wife called me to tell me that I had created a monster in her calm and pleasant husband and that her "new" husband was intolerable, fighting with his carpool, and about to kill their neighbors. Giving these patients a torrent of testosterone also enlarged their prostates and increased their propensity for atherosclerotic heart disease, as fat levels in the body (total cholesterol) and high-density lipoproteins (good cholesterol) are overly sensitive to levels of hormones. Still, we look at these treatments, because there are effects and even through the misfires the answers might be out there for some of our biggest problems.

Today, research on estrogen and other hormones centers around the effects that they have not only on immunity, but also on conditions like cancer, blood clotting, and heart disease, and my patients and millions of others are living laboratories to what the future may reveal. We have found that estrogen can modulate your T cell activity, turning your immune system's rheostat up or down. The likely mechanisms are that the hormones affect the genes that provoke the disease which is the way hormones work for other things such as raising blood sugar or making your thyroid overactive.

There might be something going on with the thymus gland, too, which plays a role in immunity, autoimmunity, and aging. As a person ages after puberty, the thymus gland—the city hall of your immune system where the T cells are sorted out and get their marching orders about self or nonself during a person's development—shrinks in response to testosterone or male hormone in both men and women. All this shrinkage occurs after puberty as a normal process because of hormonal shifts. But if there is an extra dose of estrogen or the man or woman lacks testosterone, the thymus gland continues to stay right below the thyroid in the neck, abnormally large in size. This can be imperceptible for many years. This is the case with Klinefelter patients, women who are hyper-estrogenized for reasons that are not clear, males who are called hypogonadal and lack levels of male hormone, and patients with an autoimmune and neuromuscular disorder called myasthenia gravis or "grave muscular weakness," which causes weakness and rapid fatigue of muscles you normally control to breathe and move.

Or consider polycystic ovary syndrome (PCOS), a common hormonal disorder in women. PCOS is associated with dramatic rises and falls of both estrogen and androgen levels. As these hormones ebb and flow, guided by the patient's ovary and its cysts, she experiences a wash of male hormones with beard growth and high blood sugars for a few weeks. That is followed by a wave of estrogen with the loss of the beard, soft skin, and the recurrence of the menses (blood and other discharge from menstruation) for several weeks. One of my PCOS patients called these phases "Harriet" (more estrogen) versus "Harry" (more androgen). In her Harriet phase, she had a concurrent autoimmune attack with pain, fever, and weakness, which implicated her estrogens. During her Harry phase, she was symptom-free, but she had sugar problems and high blood pressure. This corresponds with evidence that men with strong levels of testosterone are impervious to autoimmune devastation. But even then, there are exceptions, as some men with normal male hormones become extremely ill with forms of autoimmune disease that defy explanation.

PCOS brings us back to the idea that the root of the problems might have more to do with the sex chromosomes and epigenetics than with sex hormones. After all, we know being a woman biologically makes you vulnerable to autoimmune diseases. We also know male hormones protect men from immune devastation in most cases, yet not after severe infections like COVID-19. These exceptions are not understood, nor is the fact that some men, despite normal levels of male hormone, get autoimmune diseases that are much worse than the disease seen in women. In fact, men with the worst rheumatoid arthritis or lupus have normal levels of male hormone. Replenishment of hormones does nothing to change the symptoms of the disease.

In the immortal words of the King of Siam in the musical *The King and I*, "'Tis a puzzlement." Simply put, what we have today is clues as to how female and male hormones intensify or ameliorate the symptoms of autoimmune disease and theories of the crime but no arrests. The solving of this mystery has major implications for immunity strong.

DR. BOB SAYS

There is a difference between biological men and women when it comes to the presentation of disease. For example, most autoimmune diseases predominate in women after puberty. This means that hormones play a role, but not enough to cause disease. So, the cause remains a mystery for medicine and science.

SO, WHAT ABOUT GENDER?

Let me repeat something I just said: Being a woman *biologically* makes you vulnerable to autoimmune disease. When we speak of someone's gender, we are not talking about biological determination but about social and cultural constructs. No matter what gender you express, your cells are still male or female. That doesn't mean gender expression can't have an impact on immunity outside of biological sex. There is also no question that behavioral changes like mood shifts, depression, aggression, and even psychoses are affected by the metabolism of hormones, and many transgender people suffer from these conditions. (The suicide rate for transgender people is ten times the national rate, which undoubtably reflects public prejudice against transgender people that affects their living conditions and day-to-day lives and most likely contributes to that suicide rate.) For example, as we learned in Chapter 3, the release of non sex hormones like oxytocin or the "love hormone" can affect immunity. If people identifying, dressing, and behaving in the world opposite the biological sex they were born makes them happy like a hug, which would serve anyone well, then those actions can positively affect their biological soul with the release of oxytocin. But none of these actions are of concern when it comes to biological sex and sex hormones and chromosomes. This is not a judgment on any person's identity, choice, or feeling, but a pure statement of biology.

What *does* obfuscate the body's two-party sex system and has drastic immunological effects is injecting hormones to change gender expression (to produce breasts, facial and body hair, or other characteristics which are not part of their biological inheritance at birth). In addition, choosing gender affirmation surgery (what we used to mislabel a sex change operation as it does not change a patient's biological sex) to alter one's external appearance from the biological sex that is baked into your genetic barcode may also have unintended epigenetic consequences that result from too much estrogen or too little androgen.

Epigenetics is controlled by sex steroids or hormones like estrogens in women and androgens in men. An individual who wishes to change their biological sex will have epigenetic effects from the use of hormones in an effort to change the way they appear to others. I saw this when I gave my Klinefelter patients testosterone to alter their immune responses. The effects were dramatic and not welcome by the patient or their loved ones; the physical effects like big feet and thick necks never changed, but the behavioral aggression of the alpha male (if such exists) was transient and stopped once the extra hormone was removed. We are still learning about these effects of the sex hormone epigenetics—including mental illness, suicidality, and depression—on the biological soul. What we do know is all this metabolic change is inextricably linked to your sex hormones—and possibly shifts in your immune system.

As we learned in the previous chapters of this book, substances that are placed in the body, like alcohol or nicotine, alter hormone metabolism and likely epigenetics, or a change in the way genes express themselves without changing the nature of the DNA. Alcohol and nicotine and more than likely tars from tobacco affect mitochondrial function and the enzymes within the cells called microsomes. These chemicals that you choose to ingest induce or lower your microsome's activity. If you are an alcoholic, your liver is primed, and the enzymes are induced unless you overdo it and wind up with alcoholic hepatitis or cirrhosis. You know when your doctor writes a prescription and the label says, "Do not drink grapefruit juice with this drug"? It means that the grapefruit juice will turn your enzymes in the cell down or compete with them and the drug would be inactivated. There are thousands of such interactions, and many are with hormones that affect the immune system.

Now, imagine injecting those hormones into your body. As we covered in Chapter 9, hormones have major epigenetic effects on the chromosomes of cells. This means that hormonal imprinting because of epigenetics has effects, albeit temporary, on the behavior of cells in every organ, but particularly the immune system. Scientists agree that this is most likely the way that sex hormones affect the immune system. Female hormones are metabolized differently in women, women who are pregnant, men, and men with the extra sex chromosome (XXY) that have immune diseases. I have also reviewed several scientific studies that have noted instances where injection of estrogen into a male body to change the male phenotype into that of a female have resulted in autoimmune disease. The belief is that the one X chromosome in that male was activated to produce the abnormality upon injection of large doses of estrogen.

It is the feeling of most endocrine biochemists that hormones act on the immune system epigenetically or outside of the Mendelian genetics or regular inheritance. As a result, it is especially important that anyone changing their gender realize that they might uncover a hidden susceptibility to immune disease.

PREGNANCY AND THE IMMUNE SYSTEM

No matter how you identify or feel about sex and gender, we all came into the world the same way. From fertilization of the egg to birth, pregnancy is an immunologic tour de force which protects an expectant mother through the usual nausea, anxiety, and stress. I liken it to a nine-month-long symphony performed by hundreds of musicians and choir members working tirelessly together. I marvel at the way pregnancy represses a woman's normal cell reactivity or perceived violation of her immune response in her body so that fetal cells can increase, and her baby can grow. That's because the baby in her womb is an infringement on the rules of the immune system; it contains half of the genome of the father and thus has its own genetic makeup distinct from the mother. The fact that the baby has a genetic dissimilarity is actually good and an immunological advantage. If the baby were genetically related to both mother and father (as in some closed societies or as a result of incestuous comingling), the baby would be likely be miscarried or born with severe birth defects and die an early death.

Through a constant series of complex, delicate, and meticulous interactions involving cytokines and too many cells to count, the mother's immune system plays a role in all three phases of the pregnancy process: inflammation (to allow implantation), anti-inflammation (to allow for gestation), and inflammation again (to allow birth to occur). The immunogenetics of the maternal-fetal interface, which is where the mother's circulation and the baby's circulation come together, protect the baby. This is a process so beautiful and immunologically complex and profound that the mother needs to grow a new organ to bring it all together: the placenta—the nourishing fetal docking station a mother grows within her uterus.

The main players in the remodeling that goes on to make room for and grow the placenta and fetus are the cells and molecules of the immune system. Without this remodeling, there can be no interface between the baby and the mother for the exchange of oxygen and nutrients (which is what happens in many stillbirths).

Cells invade the uterine lining, new vessels are formed, and layers of protection for the baby are produced. The cells that predominate during the early stages are called, perhaps surprisingly, killer cells, which are cells derived from the uterine tissues and make up 70 percent of the lymphocytes that surround the fertilized egg. In contrast to the natural killer T cells in the rest of the mother's body, however, these killer cells are weaker and have different roles. They are the source of cytokines that make blood vessels grow and other chemicals that allow the placenta to develop like *metalloproteinases*. Metalloproteinases are interesting chemicals with curious properties. They are part of a family of enzymes that break down proteins between cells and vital to the remodeling that goes on in the placenta to allow a baby to grow peacefully. Like many enzymes, they need zinc and calcium to work properly, which is where the enzyme class gets its name.

While there is a lack of fetal antigen expression, macrophages or antigen-presenting cells watch over the maternal-fetal boundary like a sophisticated border patrol, looking at everything that comes in and out of the fetal fluids and blood. They also eat the leftovers of cells that implode (*apoptosis*) while the egg is burrowing into the wall of the uterus. T lymphocytes or helper cells (specifically the T helper 2 cells) of both the innate and adaptive immune system are also incorporated into the pregnancy process not only at the maternal-fetal border but also throughout the system of the mother. This T helper cell population goes into anti-inflammatory mode, meaning that their numbers increase to ensure the fetal "programming" (the way that the baby will develop after birth) is correct and that the development of the fetus goes well for all nine months.

While all this programming is happening inside the mother, maternal immune stimulation during pregnancy from the outside acts as an environmental risk factor to that programming and thus her baby's brain and immune system development after birth. A mother can be infected during pregnancy with a variety of organisms that will affect the outcome of the baby; outcomes that can include schizophrenia, autism, and other neurodevelopmental conditions. My concern as a doctor is caring for those who do not live in a nurturing environment for the baby in utero. Many of the abnormalities found in children result from an imbalance brought on by the conditions of and external influences on the mother's life during pregnancy. Alcohol consumption, smoking, doing drugs (both illicit and over-the-counter), and even extreme stress affects the mother, can alter the fine immune balance during pregnancy, and will result in a baby whose fetal programming is off or disturbed. As we learn more about pregnancy and immunity, it is imperative that we take particular care to make sure that the mother avoids these influences, has guaranteed nutrition, and receives vaccinations against influenza, tetanus, diphtheria, pertussis, and other more urgent conditions like COVID-19, as infection during gestation is a major risk for the fetus.

While all this programming is going on, sex and other hormones play a role in a healthy pregnancy, too. Prolactin, the milk producing hormone and cytokine that comes from the pituitary gland, is influential during this time. As the mother's immune system deals with multiple glandular and overall bodily changes, it is held stable by prolactin, which stimulates the immune system and allows B cells, which react with a person's own organs, to escape due process. In addition, prolactin increases the production of antibodies, helps to complete T cell development, and decisively shifts the population of T cells from a nasty inflammatory series of cells to ones which promote tolerance, inhibiting the normal responses of killer lymphocytes during pregnancy. Meanwhile, sex hormone steroids like progesterone, estrogen, and human chorionic gonadotrophin provide for a healthy placenta and fetus. These hormones are a big reason for the shift of T cells from T helper 1 to T helper 2 cells and give the pregnancy the proper codes for the cytokines to communicate. This profile changes from T helper 2 to T helper 1 cells at the time of labor as T helper 1 cells produce an inflammatory profile, which assists the mother with labor and takes care of the placental remnants at birth.

Sex hormone metabolism, the effects of hormones on cells, the propensity for immune disease in either immune system political party (man or woman), the amazing power of hormones on the expression of genes, the wonders of hormone regulation and immunity; all of this and more shows you how everything comes full circle in this chapter as sex hormones play amazing roles in reproduction, not just sex status and immune homeostasis. Men and women are marvels to behold, but pregnant women show the expansive wonders of our biological soul for the future of the human race.

DR. BOB SAYS

Hormones and epigenetics are operatives in the cause of female predominant diseases. Much has to do with the fine-tuned immune systems of women, who by design have to carry an infant to term. But it is more than that. The secrets lie in the sex chromosomes. Over time, the mystery of pregnancy might lend us a clue. After all, it is a miracle that most babies are born normal and survive the biology and behaviors of their mothers.

10 Pain and Fatigue
The Frontier of the Brain–Immune System Connection

Marty came to my clinic six months after contracting COVID-19. At the outset of the infection, his symptoms were a nagging dry cough, shortness of breath, loss of taste and smell, and severe aches that did not respond to traditional anti-inflammatory drugs like Advil. As a result, he had spent most of the first week in bed until all but his cough disappeared. That cough had been accompanied by a shortness of breath that came and went and made climbing the single flight of stairs to his apartment difficult. By then, however, Marty was just glad that he had no reason to go to the hospital. Plus, he worked from home as a computer programmer, so he didn't need to climb those stairs much. He felt like he was on the road to recovery.

A few weeks later, Marty's cough and shortness of breath disappeared, but he was back in my office. He told me he "just did not have a lot of energy." He sat at his desk each day but was barely productive and often unable to function and keep things straight. Before the coronavirus infection, he could sleep four or five hours and night and be fine. Now, he told me, he slept upwards of ten hours a night and none of it was restful. To me, he looked listless.

Many of us learned more than we ever had about the immune system during the COVID-19 pandemic, but perhaps the biggest education—even to us doctors—was just how long it can take to resolve the symptoms of the infection and how varied those symptoms can be. To be sure, symptoms take time to resolve in many infections, and there are hundreds of viruses out there that could be responsible for conditions like Marty's. If you get a viral infection like influenza or COVID-19, you will have symptoms that are peripheral (sneezing, coughing), which mostly resolve themselves after a few weeks or more, and those that are neurologic (headache, muscle pain) that can take longer to disappear. In patients who are quite ill, fever, fatigue, weakness, loss of appetite, foggy thinking, and that "sick feeling" are not uncommon. But when neurologic symptoms endure in Marty and others for months or years after the initial infection without any additional inflammation, they could be suffering from what we call long-haul syndrome (or PASC, Post-Acute Sequelae of SARS-CoV-2 infection).

Understanding what causes pain without other symptoms of immune dysfunction is an ongoing problem for scientists and physicians. The sheer volume of long-haul COVID-19 patients could open the door to a brain–immune system connection for chronic disorders like chronic fatigue syndrome and fibromyalgia that have been dismissed by physicians as "all in your head." Don't get me wrong: I agree. They *are* in your head, just not *all*. I believe there is a mind-body connection at work and understanding what this means on the frontier of immunology is the subject of this chapter.

THE LONG HAUL OF PAIN AND FATIGUE

Marty was a classic case in which the typical markers of inflammation are not evident after an infection event. Remember what we learned in Chapter 6: Inflammation—characterized by swelling, redness, and pain—is your immune system reacting to a criminal invasion. Your first responders head to the scene of the crime with a flow of cells to cordon off the scene, arrest the invader, and carry it to the Alcatraz of the spleen or lymph node for destruction. The pain you experience is a sign of your biological soul serving you well. But in patients like Marty, the inflammation is long gone. Just like chronic pain conditions that make patients feel horrible, there is no inflammation, so it seems to the doctor that there is nothing to treat.

Thus begins a patient's long haul through neurologic symptoms like brain fog, headache, numbness and tingling of the hands and feet, loss of taste and smell, muscle pain, and dizziness, all of which were common in long-haul COVID-19 patients. The COVID-19 virus appears to be neurotrophic, meaning it prefers to attack nerves and the brain. A study out of the United Kingdom confirmed observations of profound neurologic disability and found irreversible neurologic damage to the brains of many patients during and after COVID-19 infection and that those who lost their senses of taste and smell are lucky to have them return. All these symptoms are exhausting and depressing—and heartbreaking to witness—which is why Marty and other long-haul patients complain of fatigue. These two very debilitating complications of disease are felt by most people—including doctors like me—to be both frustrating and complex. Every doctor in practice had seen patients complaining of fatigue before COVID-19. I'd seen it countless times in patients with autoimmune diseases like rheumatoid arthritis, multiple sclerosis, lupus, and any condition where there is chronic inflammation. But what about noninflammatory conditions? That pain and fatigue is more difficult for doctors like me to understand.

Patients with these pain syndromes feel as though they have inflammation but show no signs of swelling or redness. They may feel that medication will take away the pain as it would with conditions like arthritis or muscle disease, but the pain and discomfort are general and unresponsive to anti-inflammatory drugs of any kind. The few drugs that we possess to remove the pain act on the central nervous system in ways we do not fully understand, and there is no medication that will remove the pain successfully, let alone the chronic fatigue. This could be one of the great mysteries of medicine, or an immunological "sleight of hand," in which the true mechanisms of pain come from the brain and not the site of the pain at all. It is as if the processes of inflammation and immune response are undermined by a stealthy mind-body connection that has been corrupted.

Parkinson's disease, post-polio syndrome, and stroke are examples of neurologic conditions with no clear inflammatory component in which fatigue is not only common but incredibly debilitating. Chronic fatigue is also found in cancer patients, particularly those undergoing chemotherapy where proinflammatory cytokines used to mitigate side effects might be the culprits. These proinflammatory cytokines are probably in the brain and possibly connected to long-haul syndrome with COVID-19, which makes these cytokines erupt in some patients' brains. So, am I saying all these diseases are immune diseases or immunologically linked? Maybe they are, but science has not unraveled these complex symptoms in relation to the biological soul. But COVID-19 long-haul patients have raised the stakes considerably for finding a solution.

Even a hint of a solution will be important for the millions of people suffering from fibromyalgia (a disorder that causes widespread chronic muscle soreness and tenderness) and chronic fatigue syndrome (which is also called myalgic encephalomyelitis and causes profound and chronic fatigue and pain as well as sleep problems). Emanating from the brain but manifested in the arms, legs, and torso, these conditions are associated with immune disease through mechanisms that remain puzzling. Both are noninflammatory conditions that are difficult to assign blame for. What is clear is they are the source of endless discomfort. With no response from steroids or anti-inflammatory medicines, they haunt patients with unrelenting pain and sleep deprivation. They are crippling and "life stealing" conditions as they destroy patients' quality of life in the process.

Simply put, it can be pure hell.

It is complex and interesting where fatigue and pain come together in my opinion, and the approach to these pain and fatigue syndromes should be explored with a mind-body connection. There is some data to support the idea that chronic fatigue and fibromyalgia are the residua of a viral infection in some patients, especially fibromyalgia, which often accompanies autoimmune disease and is thus more common to women. There is also evidence the possible reasons for this unrelenting pain and extreme fatigue could be a problem with cellular communication and the effects of cytokines in the brain. Those are just some of the reasons I believe these disorders are biologically mediated pain syndromes that exist in the patient's brain but manifest themselves in the peripheral tissues like muscles and ligaments and even the bowel as irritable bowel syndrome.

The problem is physicians—really good and qualified physicians—have leaned and continue to lean only toward the behavior side of things when it comes to fibromyalgia (less so with chronic fatigue syndrome). They don't see this condition as anything but behavioral, forcing patients suffering from this hell of chronic pain and fatigue out of the physician's office and onto the psychiatrist's couch. But with so many people, especially women, complaining about chronic pain and fatigue—sleepless and too uncomfortable and exhausted to work, play with their kids, cook, and do ordinary tasks—I think we owe at least a consideration of other approaches.

My hypothesis is the culprits are a mix of genetics, immune system function, personality, and/or psychological traits. I also believe there could be inflammation without inflammation, namely inflammation in the brain without classic symptoms like fever or pain beyond a mild headache or migraine, and that this is why traditional anti-inflammatory meds don't work. Let's break and think about what I mean with a deeper dive into the mind-body connection and then examine those two frustrating, mysterious, and oft-dismissed conditions: chronic fatigue syndrome and fibromyalgia.

DR. BOB SAYS

The chronic pain and fatigue produced by diseases like fibromyalgia and chronic fatigue syndrome are immune-related and connected to the terrible consequences of a viral or bacterial infection or related in some way to autoimmunity. Before COVID-19, patients (mostly women) who suffered from these diseases were treated in a psychiatrist's couch, not a doctor's office.

THE MIND-BODY CONNECTION TO IMMUNITY, PAIN, AND FATIGUE

Okay, get ready; this is "heady" stuff! While your immune system and brain organ systems maintain your homeostasis, your brain tries to run the show in your body. From behavior to immune response, it influences every relationship, including the communication between the immune system and the peripheral nervous system. Certain aspects of this brain-body connection are clear, such as the facts that neurons are integral components of your immune system and that your immune system relies on reflex nerve circuits which influence cells within the bloodstream.

Born in the brain, neurons or nerve cells in the central nervous system transmit impulses through electrical and chemical signals that carry information throughout your body and coordinate the function of human life. Sensory nerve cells are present on the front line of all our host defenses and like the cells we call macrophages or antigen-presenting cells, nerve cells interact directly with inflammatory products of the viruses, bacteria, parasites, and subsequently you, the host. In fact, the neural relationships with the blood cells of the immune system allow a rapid response to many threats to it. This is in effect the internet of the body, and it relies on *action potentials*, the body's electric system which is the basis for electrical signaling in those neurons, to run.

Action potentials of the nervous system is the immune system's quick way of transmitting information, above and beyond that of cytokines and chemokines. To refresh your memory, your cells must communicate prior to going to the scene of an inflammatory event. To coordinate this response, your immune system has a communication network called the biological regulatory system, which is composed of a pair of powerful chemicals: cytokines (which tell cells what to do) and chemokines (which tell cells where to go). These chemicals are produced throughout the body and provide quick and long-lasting innate and adaptive response. But when an even faster response is needed to major infection or injury, like a severe burn to a raging pneumonia from a virus and other traumatic invasions and events, your innate response counts on the nerve-immune system connection and the cytokines released by nerve cells.

Your immune system's sensory and motor nerve connections are the fundamental components of this simple but powerful inflammatory reflex. They communicate in milliseconds that something terrible has happened and the brain should respond accordingly, making them crucial in the defense against infection and major factors in distinguishing self from nonself. Your thymus and lymph nodes, liver, spleen, and bowel are all richly supplied with nerves capable of transmitting information to and from the nervous system to regulate the activity of white blood cells during the exposure of those cells to infectious agents and other antigens or because of major injuries to the body.

This inflammatory reflex is the ultimate collaboration of your immune system and nerve cells. On the surface of lymphocytes and other kinds of white cells within the immune system are receptors for alpha- and beta-adrenergic responses, which tell these cells how to behave and where to proceed. Basically, this is a response of the immune cells to hormones produced by the nervous system like cortisone or other substances that come from the pituitary gland at the base of the brain and the conductor of your glandular orchestra. Antibody and cellular responses within the immune system depend heavily on the nervous system's regulation of neural hormones, which are directed by the brain. Add to it the hormone effects and you have a master work of responsiveness, like a symphony orchestra working together to create great music.[1]

There are various parts of our bodies that showcase this neuroimmune inflammatory reflex, indicating that within the bloodstream the cells of the immune system share the defense of the body with the nervous system and how the nervous system and the lymphocyte-macrophage nexus can detect subtle changes in the body's environment. Macrophages respond to invasions by producing a variety of cytokines and other mediators, and neurons respond by producing action potentials. So, both neurons and macrophages share the responsibility to protect us from intrusions, and the innate immune system is up front with a remarkable defense.

For example, in your gut or bowel biome with its billions of bacteria, the enteric neural reflex involves macrophages or antigen-presenting cells being stratified in the layers of the intestinal wall, protecting it from dangerous scavenging bacteria and other foreign antigens like parasites. This finely tuned protective mechanism prevents damage to the bowel wall from chronic inflammation. In the lung, cytokines and chemokines work to protect the exchange of oxygen and CO_2, and there is a delicate balance similar to the one in your bowel. These are easily disrupted by inflammation from viruses or bacteria, or micro clotting as a result of inflammation. When increased cytokines and cells accumulate in allergic or viral induced lung inflammation, specific cytokines are released by activated immune cells and a variety of lymphocytes respond to the lung, amplifying the inflammatory response. This was very common in COVID-19 infections and was part of the long-haul syndrome, in which patients could not breathe without oxygen six months or more after their infections.

---

[1] All of your director hormones come from the pituitary gland. I can remember a professor of mine referring to the pituitary gland as the conductor of the endocrine system "orchestra," which the system made up of the glands within your body like the adrenal, thyroid, and pituitary.

Recent research into this nerve-immune connection has led to a potential cure (not just treatment) for the most common auto-immune disease: rheumatoid arthritis. Called e-immunotherapy, the therapy takes advantage of the relationship between auto-immune disease, inflammation, and the nervous system. It uses electrical pulse sequences delivered via specially designed earbuds that target and stimulate the cholinergic anti-inflammatory pathway. In other words, the ear buds allow the brain to regulate immune function through the ear. Even in the research phase, the results look impressive: 53 percent of the patients wearing the device showed a reduction in signs and symptoms of rheumatoid arthritis.

Clearly, mind over matter begins here, as the brain can regulate immunity in ways never imagined. Its cytokines, such as TNF alpha, interleukin 1 (IL-1), IL-6, IL-12, and IL-17, are proinflammatory and important players in the inflammatory response for all infections. These cytokines are also at the biological origin of fatigue, specifically a flood of them in response to an innate response by the immune system to a catastrophic event. I like what Dr. Avindra Nath, clinical director of the National Institute of Neurological Disorders and Stroke at the National Institutes of Health, said in a December 2020 National Institutes of Health study referenced in the *New England Journal of Medicine*: "When fighting a pathogen, the immune system sometimes conducts a very precise and surgical attack, working like a guided missile," but when that approach fails, it can begin "carpet bombing," which is more difficult to control, because it is persistent immune activation.

Interleukin 1 (IL-1), a very potent cytokine in the body, is one of the most thoroughly investigated cytokines and acts in the brain to mediate lack of appetite, withdrawal in response to fear, and is believed to be a major player in all the inflammation and "sickness behavior" (that sick feeling Marty had). Most of us have experienced these proinflammatory cytokines when we get a severe cold, the flu, COVID-19, or any major injury that involves inflammation and leads to sickness behavior symptoms, such as inability to function or need to sleep (i.e., fatigue). In humans, the intravenous administration of IL-1 beta leads to fatigue, fever, chills, and headaches. Administration of a drug that is an IL-1 receptor antagonist or anti-inflammatory produces rapid and profound relief of fatigue.

The cytokine IL-6 also does a lot of things to the brain. IL-6 is able to cross the blood-brain barrier and enter the brain. If you recall from Chapter 2, microglia, along with astrocytes, are the two neurologic cells that wear first responder badges in the brain. In other words, they are neuronal but also immunological. They are the brain's internal immune cells and like an elite corps of cells with special privileges are dedicated to protecting your brain from infection (and also might allow B cells and T cells to come in). I see them as a kind of praetorian guard of the brain, capable of mediating the behavior of illness and changing the nerve status of the host.

When elevated levels of IL-6 cross the blood-brain barrier, they can activate the microglia cells in the brain, causing extreme fatigue. Therefore, patients with lupus and rheumatoid arthritis who have elevated levels of IL-6 and are given blocking agents report significant relief from tiredness and fatigue. It is also why during COVID-19 we routinely measured Il-6 levels in a COVID patient's blood and sometimes tried to lower the levels of IL-6 in those who were critically ill in the hope of saving their lives as it is a big mediator of inflammation in the lungs as well.

The mystery of how all of this works is just beginning to be understood, but we can conclude from all I have covered plus animal experiments[2] and observations of people who have had severe infections that it is the messengers of the immune system like IL-1 and IL-6, as well as TNF (tumor necrosis factor) and C-reactive proteins, that are associated with proinflammatory conditions. But that won't help my patients who suffer from fibromyalgia and chronic fatigue syndrome. Those disorders have no such markers

---

[2] Pro-inflammatory cytokines from studies in animal brains during infectious events cause a behavioral response called *sickness behavior*, characterized by drowsiness, loss of appetite, decreased activity, and withdrawal from social interactions.

but might be the result of inflammation within the brain as a result of cytokine activity that is not evident. Perhaps much or all of it is happening in the brain, and we have little access to this privileged site.

> **DR. BOB SAYS**
>
> Your brain and the immune system work together, but I suspect that the immune system takes orders from the brain on most occasions through the "internet" of the immune system: your nervous system, with which the immune system has direct contact.

FIBROMYALGIA

Moira, a married woman of 32, came to me on a referral from her primary care physician. She had been treated for Sjogren's syndrome. Moira not only had the typical dry mouth and eyes from this "desert syndrome," but her mucous membranes like those around her vagina were parched, making sexual relations with her husband impossible. She was placed on a high dose of corticosteroid to control the symptoms, and it did. But it did nothing for her pain. She found it difficult if not impossible to take care of her three-year-old and do work around the house. She still could not even think of having a relationship with her husband. Moira's marriage was falling apart because of this feeling of being in constant pain and the resulting exhaustion from a lack of sleep. Since no over-the-counter medications helped her pain, she had been placed on large doses of prednisone to treat her condition, which did nothing but make her gain weight. When we examined her, we looked for signs of inflammation and found nothing. We, too, began to believe that Moira was crazy, anxious, or both. But if she was either of those things it was *because* of her condition, not the condition itself.

Moira is one of many millions of young women with fibromyalgia, one of the most vexing conditions physicians see. It is the disorder where fatigue and pain come together. Let me say it one more time: Fibromyalgia is a real condition, not a behavioral condition or a psychiatric illness. It is a biologically mediated pain syndrome that exists in the patient's brain but manifests itself in the peripheral tissues like muscle and ligaments and even the bowel as irritable bowel syndrome. The condition often accompanies autoimmune diseases—which is why more women than men are affected by it—or occasionally happens by itself. Patients with this condition also have sleep disturbances and rarely get a good night's sleep. Some have a condition called brain fog where they find it difficult to recall things. Sound familiar? It is precisely what is seen in many long-haul COVID-19 patients.

Fibromyalgia is difficult to treat and even more difficult to diagnose. Diseases like fibromyalgia might be inflammatory conditions limited to the brain, wherein the usual markers are not evident, because it is centrally mediated pain. That's why so many doctors think these patients are crazy. They are looking for traditional signs of inflammation like elevated white cell counts, fever, C-reactive proteins, sedimentation rate ... but it is not traditional inflammation, meaning that it is likely that all inflammation might not produce redness, fever, soreness, and debilitation. The only place psychology comes in is the way patients like Moira manage the pain and fatigue, which has a major effect on their presentation. For example, I can diagnose it by pressing specific tender points on the body that all the patients with fibromyalgia have. But there is *no* inflammation at the sites where these patients go, "Ow!" The ow is coming from their brains. But then I will press a tip of the finger, which is not one of the tender points specific to fibromyalgia, and the patient to cooperate will say, "Ow!" Because they want to impress me that they are hurting all over and desperately need someone to believe them after being told it was just in their head.

While doctors seeing patients struggle with how to deal with millions of fibromyalgia patients, research is being done to help them. Dr. Jarred Younger, who leads the Neuroinflammation, Pain and Fatigue Laboratory at the University of Birmingham in

Alabama, believes the brain's microglial cells are responsible for fibromyalgia. When these cells become hypermobile, the rush of proinflammatory cytokines suppress dopamine, a particularly important chemical that is involved in the function of your nerve cells and your mood. Younger's theory is that an event like an infection from a virus causes the microglial cells to enter this dangerous state and causes patients to become overly sensitive when they enter a state of chronic inflammation.

If we accept Younger's belief and theory that fibromyalgia exists primarily as a pathologic state in the brain, an organ that has only privileged access to many medications, we can understand why standard analgesics and anti-inflammatories have no effect on the microglial cells. Younger believes that drugs like quercetin and curcumin (both in clinical trials as I write this) could influence the microglial population of the brain. By extension, drugs that suppress microglia like naltrexone and minocycline among others also could influence the microglial cells and control this debilitating condition. Many investigators, including me, are pursuing a similar path, using low-dose naltrexone to treat fibromyalgia with modest success.

In other work being done, there are doctors who believe that mitochondria—the prehistoric bacterial energy factories of your cells—are to blame for, or at least are involved in, the cause of fibromyalgia as well as chronic fatigue syndrome, as disturbances of mitochondrial function can cause a reduction of energy and energy consumption. Right away, this intrigues me since we only get our mitochondria from our mothers (spermatozoa do not have it) and women are disproportionately affected by these diseases.

Even though they were bacteria at some point in our evolution, mitochondria are not considered part of our biome but because they were free living bacteria millions of years ago. But maybe they should be. Mitochondria are intracellular organelles that retain multiple features of their bacterial ancestry that only exist in the egg or oocyte before fertilization and are given to us by our mothers. They are involved in the regulation of both macrophages and T cells of the immune system and can encourage either heightened or deficient immune responses. There can be deficiencies of natural killer T cells, downregulation of innate immune activity, and weakened B cell receptor expression, all of which have significant effects on the average person's immune response.

Inflammatory reactions and activation of the innate and adaptive immune responses can be triggered by alteration of mitochondrial functions. (The term used by many people is oxidative stress.) The late Dr. Lewis Thomas, whose writing clarifying the mysteries of biology made him renowned as a poet-philosopher of medicine, always thought that mitochondria had a special place in regulating illness. Researchers have looked for years at mitochondria particularly in nerve cells as a possible cause of multiple sclerosis that manifests without a lot of inflammation. Similar claims have been made by others about all kinds of diseases that manifest without inflammation. For example, in autoimmune diseases of the eye, antiretinal antibodies can be found in the absence of inflammation.

For sure, there are also diseases that are specific to mitochondria that don't involve chronic fatigue, which means the mystery continues. What this means for now is there is evidence that inflammation can happen in parts of the body as a result of the immune system's subtle effects in our brains. This is very good news for patients with chronic fatigue syndrome who were also dismissed as crazy for well over a century.

DR. BOB SAYS

Fibromyalgia is a horrible immune-related disease that wreaks havoc on people and families and is more common than doctors would like. It is associated with infections and autoimmune diseases, but there are no signs of peripheral inflammation in blood tests, just subjective complaints that are reproduced from patient to patient.

CHRONIC FATIGUE SYNDROME

Most medical history traces chronic fatigue syndrome back to George Miller Beard, an American neurologist who coined the term *neurasthenia* in the nineteenth century to describe a disease the symptoms of which included fatigue, anxiety, headache, and depression. History has since been unkind to neurasthenia, which came to be seen as a "neurotic disorder" (which is still its classification by the World Health Organization). History has been more kind to the study of the profound and chronic fatigue and pain as well as sleep problems first noted by Beard. Eventually the Centers for Disease Control (CDC) coined the term *chronic fatigue syndrome* in 1987. Later, *myalgic encephalomyelitis* was added to the name and the syndrome became known in medicine as ME/CFS.

The CDC's 1994 definition (clinically evaluated, unexplained, persistent, or relapsing chronic fatigue) and diagnostic criteria (not a lifelong condition, not the result of ongoing exertion, not alleviated by rest, substantial effect on work/school, social, and/or personal activities) of ME/CFS remain the most common worldwide. Because of this widely accepted definition and diagnostic criteria, we have better statistics on ME/CFS: It largely affects young people between the ages of 29 and 45 years; women represent 75 to 90 percent of those affected; and about 200,000 new cases are diagnosed each year. While the scientific literature deals with many different subtypes of chronic fatigue syndrome, it basically identifies and validates consistent biomarkers for an objective diagnosis. Studies have shown that ME/CFS patients have deficiencies in major cell types of the innate immune system, including extreme antiviral cytotoxic or natural killer T cells and reduced receptor expression on B cells. In other words, immune deficiencies are found in this condition. And, blessedly, in a 2015 report informed by a review of more than 9,000 articles from 64 years of medical literature, the National Academy of Medicine dismissed the misconception of the disease as a psychological condition.

But that doesn't mean we are any closer to understanding ME/CFS. It remains an intractable and minimally understood chronic illness of unknown cause.

When it comes to fatigue, in addition to the "carpet bombing" cytokines described before, some scientists have compared patients with chronic fatigue as reminiscent of hibernating bears. It has also been called "post-viral fatigue," although most times a virus is not identified. Personally, I have found the debility alarming, serious, and related to the immune system's goals of protecting us against all invaders. I also think epigenetic marks like methylation of histones and RNA-based modifications of gene expression is required for better understanding of the underlying disruptions in the epigenome and gene expression dynamics in chronic fatigue syndrome.

Bringing ME/CFS back to the brain, there are other interesting scenarios to consider, including the disruption of the hypothalamic pituitary adrenal axis and the release of the fight or flight hormones (like adrenalin). This response is disrupted with a muted response to fight or flight hormones in response to stress, resulting in depression in some patients with conditions like multiple sclerosis and breast cancer—patients who routinely have persistent fatigue as well. There is also an increase of oxidative stress in people with chronic inflammatory disorders such as rheumatoid arthritis and lupus.

Like I said many times in this chapter, it is a mystery, but it is one modern medicine is trying to unravel more than ever. If there is any silver lining to the COVID-19 pandemic, it is that the millions of patients suffering from long-haul symptoms have sparked new interest in ME/CFS identification and treatment. About a third of the long-haul patients I see have chronic fatigue and new pain syndromes they never had before COVID-19. It is strongly felt by investigators researching ME/CFS that the condition shares characteristics not only with these COVID-19 long-haulers, but also with fibromyalgia. Interestingly, women predominate among patients in all three situations. They share in their suffering of exhaustion that commonly worsens with physical, mental, or emotional exertion. They experience widespread muscle and joint pain, the development in many cases of high-titer autoantibodies, headaches, and many other symptoms like hair loss and lack of taste and smell. They suffer from short-term memory and concentration problems. Their profound fatigue is not relieved with sleep.

A pandemic is nothing to celebrate on any level, but insights into ME/CFS and fibromyalgia have opened up because of it and given me and many others clarity about the role viruses may play in these diseases and new frontiers for the mind-body connection when it comes to pain and fatigue.

DR. BOB SAYS

Chronic fatigue syndrome is a frustrating enigma. Like fibromyalgia, it is unrelenting and life changing—and there is only limited understanding of the condition. Immunologists like me believe it to be the result of infection and might be a cytokine issue confined to the brain.

11 Laterality, Creativity, Behavior, and the Biological Soul

In a scene from the movie *Amadeus*, Wolfgang Amadeus Mozart plays a composition backwards on the piano with his hands crossed while upside down and unable to see the keys. It is a joyous and remarkable moment, and many Mozart experts believe it could have happened. Mozart had a flair for the dramatic. He was ambidextrous. He was playing the piano blindfolded at the age of six. And by 35, he was dead, possibly of kidney disease, rheumatic fever, strep, syphilis, lupus . . . No one knows for sure, but most theories point to an infection or immune disease. There are some associations with immune dysfunction that are quite curious, including creativity, laterality, and learning problems that can be associated with immune disease and even with the presence of certain antibodies. I had wondered before if Mozart's prolific and creative genius and what killed him might be linked. Today, I am convinced of it.

This chapter explores this link between creativity, learning, and the development of our immune system. The whole concept is not without controversy, but the possibilities are too powerful to ignore. Just as epigenetics has shown that what you do and where and how you live causes changes in the way your genes work, I believe our biological soul may have no boundaries when it comes to expressions of creativity, behavior, and personality. I believe there is an inextricable link between the biological soul and behavior—between the pathological processes we have covered in this book (those caused by physical or mental disease) and brain development, laterality (a person's preference for using one side of their body over the other, like being left-handed), learning disabilities (like dyslexia or "word blindness," and dyscalculia or the inability to learn number-related concepts), creativity, and so much more. Indulge me!

INITIAL CONNECTIONS TO LATERALITY AND HANDEDNESS

It was actually a man named Fritz, not Mozart, who convinced me years before *Amadeus* hit theaters to explore this link between the immune system and laterality and creativity. Fritz was a talented 50-year-old economist who worked for the government. He came to my office on a referral from his primary care physician to treat extreme dryness to his eyes and mouth from Sjogren's syndrome. Men rarely present to my office with this or any florid autoimmune disease in middle age; they affect mostly women. Yet that was not what was most unusual about Fritz. (We treated his Sjogren's with corticosteroids to bring his tears and saliva back to near normal.) What was unusual was Fritz was not only ambidextrous but wrote and read perfectly backwards. He even *preferred* it. He spoke normally, but because he wrote backwards, his staff had to reproduce all the documents he created on a copier with a reversed mirror. Only then were they able to understand his spreadsheets, calculations, and prose.

Neither Fritz's physician nor I had ever seen anyone like Fritz, and his physician wanted to know if this had anything to do with his disease. So did I. Turns out Fritz's arrival was perfectly timed.

My exploration of laterality and handedness had started about a year before I saw Fritz. Dr. Henry G. Kunkel, my mentor at Rockefeller University, was a guest at a dinner at Harvard University in 1982 and seated with Dr. Norman Geschwind, the James Jackson Putnam Professor of Neurology at the school and a pioneering neurologist who many scientists called the best in America. Kunkel mentioned to Geschwind that autoimmune disease had been the subject of intense study in his lab. Geschwind asked whether Kunkel was interested in learning disability and laterality as it applied to autoimmune diseases. The idea of studying something as bizarre as learning disability and handedness (the tendency to use one hand over the other) with regard to autoimmunity intrigued my mentor, and when he returned from Harvard, he immediately asked me to do some exploration on learning disabilities, autoimmunity, and laterality, specifically handedness.

I was a bit surprised, as I did not know that there was an association between these things. I was even more surprised when Dr. Kunkel told me to call Geschwind. *Me*, a junior assistant professor, was going to speak to the legendary Norman Geschwind about associations between the immune system, developmental disorders, and the brain! When I called Geschwind, we arranged to meet in the bar of the Boston hotel to discuss research. I wore a red carnation in the buttonhole of my jacket so that he would recognize me, but there was no way I wouldn't recognize him and his briefcase as he approached.

Geschwind was a fast-talking man then in his early fifties, and we got right into all of the topics that day. The developmental disorders that Geschwind and his staff were concerned with at the time we met were autism, hyperactivity, stuttering, dyscalculia, developmental aphasia (or the inability to talk), and dyslexia. How these might be linked to immunology was provocative, and Geschwind and I continued to meet for years to come as associates and friends. He came to my home and enthralled my children with his ability to juggle and regaled adults with his extraordinary joke telling. We spent most of our time, however, in each other's labs.

During our enthusiastic late nights, we combined observations from two different disciplines and searched for what they might reveal. We paired neurological and immunological problems and imagined joint explanations for both. Geschwind became deeply interested in the autoimmune diseases we studied at Rockefeller like multiple sclerosis, rheumatoid arthritis, lupus, and myasthenia gravis. He was also fascinated that these diseases affected mostly females and occurred after puberty. It was an invigorating intellectual time for me—one that got even more stimulating when we did a deep dive into handedness and the differences between them. These interactions remain some of the most entertaining and interesting I have ever had and opened up my fascination with the brain and the immune system, no more so when he laid out the principles of the Geschwind-Galaburda Hypothesis.

THE GESCHWIND-GALABURDA HYPOTHESIS AND HANDEDNESS

One of the most eye-opening moments working with Geschwind was the day he opened his briefcase and handed me a questionnaire called the Edinburgh Handedness Inventory (EHI), which assesses if a person is left- or right-handed. I learned then that just asking people whether they are left- or right-handed fails to provide proof of handedness. The EHI does. It uses the questionnaire to measure your "laterality quotient" on a scale from -100 (most left-handed) to +100 (most right-handed) with perfect ambidexterity being a zero.

Personally, I never considered handedness in anything I did until I met Geschwind, but the idea that only 10 percent of the world's population is left-handed made me lean in even more to what he told me. He regaled me with stories and information. Some of them I have never been able to "prove" (like that there were many more left-handed desks at Juilliard Music School). But others were easy to confirm like the fact that Plato, Charles Darwin, Carl Sagan, and Albert Einstein were all left-handed, or that, like Mozart, Leonardo da Vinci was ambidextrous. I'll add my own observation to his: while 90 percent of the population is right-handed, five of the last nine presidents of the United States (inclusive of Joe Biden) were left-handed.

Geschwind also introduced me to Dr. Albert Galaburda, a Chilean-born neuroscientist at Harvard who studied the biological bases of developmental cognitive disorders. Among their work together in the lab, they had determined the lateralization of mice, looking for paw dominance in response to various stimuli. All the mice—and, Geschwind assured me, all animals in nature—had a paw preference. (One can study brain structure in mice more readily than in humans.) Together, based on their findings, they proposed what came to be called the Geschwind-Galaburda Hypothesis (GGH).

The GGH suggests a connection between left-handedness, learning disability, and immune disease and disorders. According to the GGH:

- Left-handed people have a higher incidence of autoimmune diseases in themselves and their immediate families than right-handers.
- Left-handers with an incidence of at least one autoimmune disease within a family were more strongly left-handed than were those with no incidents of autoimmunity.
- Testosterone levels were supportive and essential to both the immune system and the brain during fetal development.

Essentially what that last point adds is an additional hypothesis to the GGH called the "testosterone hypothesis": That male hormones affect the development of the immune system and that these conditions that appear more often in males are reflective of the levels of testosterone in the amniotic fluid of the developing fetus. Here is what Galaburda wrote about this hypothesis in 1964 in a personal communication archived at Harvard Medical School: "The observation that learning disabilities such as dyslexia and stuttering occur more often in boys suggests a hormonal effect against proper left-hemisphere development in affected individuals. Testosterone is implicated in immune development. It slows thymic growth in mice and rabbits . . . Before puberty, when testosterone effects are low in both sexes, atopic and cell mediated illnesses are more common in boys. After puberty boys are protected from clinical expression of their susceptibility and (autoimmune) disorders are more common in girls."

According to the GGH, the greater the amount of testosterone, the larger the right hemisphere of the brain and consequent left-handedness. These high levels of testosterone in the mother's womb would result in a greater incidence of left-handers by allowing enlargement of the right hemisphere of the brain, creating significant deviations from the standard distribution of brain functions, and increasing the possibility of immune dysfunction. Support was granted to the hypothesis through functional magnetic resonance imaging of the brain, a study of the ratio of the digits of in the hand, and a study of other markers to denote which hemisphere was bigger. All clearly suggested that in utero levels of testosterone could influence both cerebral and immune system development.

After spending time with Geschwind, I started to note handedness in so many areas of my work and wrote a paper that appeared in the journal *Psychoneuroendocrinology* about greater left-handedness in lupus. While visiting Harvard Medical School, I examined the brains of mice with this autoimmune disease. In their brains, there were abnormal patterns of spirals or whorls in nerve cells on one side of the skull which were also found in the human brains of patients who died prematurely and allowed scientists to autopsy their brains. These whorls reflected abnormalities of the outer layer of the brain for no apparent reason but were associated with dyslexia in humans. All the mice that had these abnormalities were left-pawed, meaning that they preferred using one paw over another to get food.

That said, Geschwind and Galaburda's work was certainly "out there" when it came to handedness and laterality. They believed the season of conception (summer or winter) is nongenetic and random and can affect hand and leg lateralization; that these changes are due to hormonal influences on the brain of the developing fetus in the womb; and that seasonal differences in seasonal rhythm would determine your handedness and more. They also suggested that a mother's male hormones or menstrual cycles during spring and early summer could play a role in the brain development of boy fetuses with genetic potential for left-handedness, meaning enlargement of the right brain hemisphere.

What is most important about the GGH is that cognitive abilities depend heavily on sex hormone concentration and their immunologic characteristics and their relationship to the lateralization of the brain. Since the articulation of the GGH, epigenetics or "imprinting" (the expression of genes, but not the changing of the genes) has been the major mechanism in the inheritance of certain transient phenomena. Geschwind and I talked at length about it, and he went on to write papers about such things as handedness in professional tennis or handedness and sexual orientation—all the result of imprinting, or what we now call *epigenetics*. Extraordinary. But like I said, it was also outside the box—perhaps too out of the box for some.

The GGH has been part of mainstream discussion on this chapter's topic for decades, with many believing the data are profound and important. But when I read some of the literature on the GGH, there are still many investigators who feel the data are not solid. For sure, some parts of the GGH have been left hanging, such as the influence of testosterone in the fetus on cerebral laterality. Geschwind was certain that high fetal testosterone concentrations exaggerated the lateralization of the brain. Brains were examined using functional transcranial Doppler ultrasonography while participants completed generation and visual short-term memory tasks. In typical fashion, left lateralization of language was more common in the high testosterone group than in the low testosterone group. Unfortunately, it is difficult to study testosterone levels in the fluid surrounding the human fetus, and the measurement of adult salivary testosterone or blood levels of the hormone doesn't give answers to the many questions posed by the Geschwind hypothesis. In fact, many investigators looking at men and women who are right- and left-handed have concluded that it is difficult to measure and requires more research.

But in other areas connecting the immune system and behavior? I believe the data is compelling and the possibilities for understanding will be of deep importance to the future of our biological soul.

DR. BOB SAYS

Though not without controversy, there is evidence that that handedness and creativity are linked to the immune system. The side of your body that is dominant is inextricably linked to immune disease because of the effect of sex steroids on the development of one side of the brain at the same time the immune system is developing.

LINKING BEHAVIOR AND IMMUNE DEVELOPMENT

So, do left-handers have specific immunological patterns? Does one or another hemisphere of the brain and the developing immune system have a role to play in immune disease when it comes to the brain and cognition? These are big questions immunologists continue to ask around Norman Geschwind's work and the GGH. Unfortunately, Geschwind died too young in 1984, but he will always be remembered for starting this conversation between the immune system and behavior, which Albert Galaburda furthered with his pioneering studies on the biological foundations of developmental dyslexia.

The GGH indicated that disorders of the immune system were more common in dyslexics and in their immediate relatives when compared to control groups. Geschwind also hypothesized that premature graying was also a characteristic of the dyslexic boys who manifested autoimmune disorders and created a model that predicted that immune disorders would be more prevalent in those who are incredibly talented, especially those who have extremely well-developed right hemisphere functions such as artists or musicians.

Geschwind and a young Irish investigator named Peter Behan showed a rate of immune disorders approximately two-and-a-half times higher in left-handed people than in right-handers. The cause of this was a high level of testosterone in the womb of the mother or an increased sensitivity of this hormone occurring at five months of pregnancy. According to Geschwind and Behan, this modified the normal development of the two cerebral hemispheres by slowing the growth of the left hemisphere and promoting the growth of the right hemisphere, thus making a person left-handed or left-dominant.

The development of the immune system and the identification of both intrinsic and extrinsic surface antigens occurs at the same time as the neurons develop in the hemispheres. Some investigators have thus concluded that there is a significant association between handedness and immunity, but what is not clear is whether this is hormonally dependent. Other recent investigations indicate that based on the genetic results, there is an increase of autoimmune conditions—multiple sclerosis, myasthenia gravis, diabetes mellitus type I, and other collagen diseases—in left-handers. There are also indications that autoimmune diseases in women during pregnancy are associated with an increased risk of learning disorder disabilities in male offspring. And a paper published from several of my colleagues showed that, when present in a mother with lupus, a specific antibody known as *anti-Ro* may result in a child with a learning disorder. (In mothers with lupus, this antibody is also associated with congenital heart block in their babies, particularly male babies.) Some investigators have noted an association between left-handedness and circulating autoantibodies in healthy young people without autoimmune diseases.

In light of all these studies and more, although unusual and provocative, the GGH deserves mention in a book on immunity, because there is no question that the immune system has a role in brain development and that the associated behavioral outcomes persist for the life of the individual. The question is simply whether it is hormonal-driven or truly immune-driven.

Think back to the two critical cell types within the brain we covered in Chapter 2: microglial cells and astrocytes. Microglial cells produce cytokines and other inflammatory molecules in response to disturbances of homeostasis in a manner similar to peripheral immune cells. Astrocytes are immunocompetent cells located throughout virtually every part of the nervous system, including the brain and the spinal cord. There is interaction between these cells via hormones, chemicals called neurotransmitters, and cytokines, the biological soul's soluble protein messengers.

Cytokines are numerous and they include tumor necrosis factor, interferon, the various interleukins 1 through 26, and all sorts of stimulating factors that come in and influence platelets, red cell development, and white cell maturation, much of which we have seen throughout the book. They also affect behaviors such as sleep, memory, and the metabolism of your brain. There are receptors for cytokines on nerve cells, microglia, and astrocytes. These receptors are in the brains of all kinds of animals, not just human beings, and undoubtedly affect the behavior of a variety of different species. For humans, neural cells also express "sickness behavior"—inducing fever and other changes within the brain like depression, foggy brain, and frequently, mental illness. It makes sense to have the behavior of an individual and the lateralization of the brain related to prominence of one hemisphere over another, but the cause is mysterious.

Still, much is known since Geschwind's early work. It is especially important to remember that immune activation of the fetus in the womb produces a robust increase in cytokine expressions at the time of any antigenic challenge. This is vital to the development of the baby's immune system because the neural immune functioning and behavior could be programmed for the life of an individual. While most of this understanding comes from animal experiments, there are real-world consequences if they prove to be true in humans. Several studies have demonstrated that immune cells such as B lymphocytes and T lymphocytes and macrophages are found in the meningeal space or sack covering the brain. They are even present at the border of the brain and the spinal cord called the blood-brain barrier. We can also say that nerve cells express genetic guided mixed histocompatibility or MHC class I molecules that regulate their connections to other nerve cells. And that microglial cells express MHC class II antigenic molecules in pathological states. So immunogenetics plays a major role regarding the brain and its development and recognition of criminals who should not be in your skull.

The startling thing to understand and digest is that the pathogenesis of neurodevelopmental disorders can depend heavily on the immune system. If we look at genome-wide association studies (GWAS) and B cell–related genes, we find that there is an association of elevated CD5 B cell levels in the blood of schizophrenic patients. This could indicate that aberrant B cell immunity is part of the cause of schizophrenia. In addition, T cells in the space around the brain called the meninges and in the blood-brain barrier, or that which we call the choroid plexus, are associated with social and cognitive behaviors. We simply do not know whether these dysfunctions are caused by deficiently developed T cells, or whether aberrations are related to the onset of many of these conditions.

In addition, many psychiatric disorders probably involve the dysregulation of immune function. Schizophrenic patients, for example, have abnormal levels of IL-1 beta, IL-6, growth factors, and all sorts of other chemicals that regulate function of the brain. Individuals suffering from these disorders have abnormal immune function and present with differences in the proteins that are critical for the nerves to interact with each other. For example, people with PTSD have increased levels of circulating inflammatory markers, increased reactivity during skin antigen tests, lower T cell counts, and an increase of overall methylation (a common epigenetic provocateur that can change expression of immune genes). There are other epigenetic marks that can be active in the brain as well, but methylation is the easiest to associate with aberrant behavior. People with autism spectrum disorders also have altered cytokine profiles in their blood, low antibody levels, and altered T cell activation.

Finally, the testosterone aspect of the GGH notes that learning disability in some people with autoimmune diseases, particularly males, happens before puberty—which is interesting because females seem to be affected more with autoimmune illness after puberty with few exceptions. Some investigators have gone to immunogenetics to explain these findings on cells that occupy treasured spaces within the brain. There are always T cells within the brain, even in the absence of disease. The immunogenetics of the brain, shared by the peripheral immune system, have genetic markers like the MHC that could affect which T cells are eliminated early in life to ensure that defective cells are removed to prevent autoimmune reactivity within the brain. The immunogenetic markers on cells like microglia and astrocytes specify which intruders are to be eliminated from the brain early on in fetal life.

Of course, there are ways around the genetic security systems in the skull. In Chapter 4 on antigens, I spoke of streptococcal infection and how it affected people with rheumatic fever, namely the concept of antigenic mimicry that allows antibodies against the strep to react with selected parts of the brain, causing an involuntary tremor called Sydenham's chorea. Some patients with Sydenham's chorea have tics, obsessive-compulsive symptoms, and ADHD. All these conditions add support to the idea that there is a common (perhaps) infectious cause to these illnesses. Or remember PANDAS, which occurs after 24 hours of a strep throat? As is the case with most behavioral illnesses involving the immune system, the psychiatrists have first dibs and begin their analysis and diagnostic labeling prior to an understanding of the pathophysiological underpinnings of what is clinically observed. Finally, in a study published in *JAMA Pediatrics* that followed more than 63,000 children born full-term in New South Wales, Australia, children whose mothers had an autoimmune disease were 30 percent more likely to develop attention deficit hyperactivity disorders, or ADHD. These data would also imply that neurodevelopmental disorders in children are related to mechanisms of autoimmune disease in the mother.

Simply put, there are no solid antibody or cell markers that would categorically suggest a biological basis for most behaviors. Sound familiar? I mention the same when I speak of fibromyalgia and chronic fatigue syndrome in the last chapter wherein patients wind up on the psychiatrist's couch.

My profession has not matured enough to deal with the cryptic, mysterious, manifestations of brain-immune phenomena. The biological soul drives behavior in many ways and places both doctors and patients on a cusp of skepticism, even though, from all I have read so far, I feel I can safely conclude that the immune system plays a crucial role in brain function. And with current scientific methods, it should be possible to discern the effects of immunity on brain maturation, and that could be important for a variety of phenomena outlined by Geschwind. These include autoimmune disease, creativity, handedness, learning disability, and perhaps even sexual preference. This is why I always ask my patients, "Are you a lefty or a righty, or can you use both hands equally?" But I really should test them with the EHI.

DR. BOB SAYS

The association of immune deficits in people with mental illness offer tantalizing clues to the origins of these diseases.

WHAT DOES THIS BRAIN–IMMUNE DEVELOPMENT CONNECTION MEAN FOR ME?

Let's take a step back. We've established that the immune system and the central nervous system are both intricate and very highly organized systems that regulate most of the human body. When the brain is developing, the immune system is developing, and both play a mutual role in each other's maturation. It is also known that in the fetus in utero, there is a wash of hormones that bathe the fetus's body and brain and greatly influence the growth of the immune system while these intricate neural networks are developing. Depending on the metabolism of hormones in the mother and the baby, this process determines which hemisphere of the brain is to be dominant. This is where handedness comes into play.

Besides recognizing that there are complexities in a baby's development, one has to wonder about the interplay of all these things. Isn't the immune system like a soul when you think of the perfect balance of all of the events during the baby's development that almost predict the future in so many ways: numerical ability, artistic creativeness, which hand or foot is dominant, allergies, autoimmunity, reading talent, stuttering, athletic ability, and many other things that the GGH hypothesized decades ago? If you believe this to be true, as I do, this is the ultimate reason your biological soul requires such reverence—not just as your protector but the basis of your future.

As you contemplate all this, put on some Mozart and look at the great works of Leonardo da Vinci. He, like my patient Fritz, was a mirror writer. He also apparently had difficulties with the written word and could have been dyslexic, which is determined by incorrect spellings that create homophonic nonwords, such as writing "rane" instead of rain. A 2019 article in the *American Journal of Medicine* argued that dyslexia could have channeled da Vinci's focus into visual thinking and maybe was the undercurrent for his brilliance and creativity. So, next time you see images of the Mona Lisa or the Vitruvian Man, I invite you to think of the power of your immune system and your brain, and how marvelous this interaction is.

DR. BOB SAYS

Like Leonardo da Vinci, you have stored in your biological soul the remnants of talents beyond your wildest imagination. One thing is certain: the mysteries of the immune system have deepened since I was introduced to this amazing association early in my career. Through the biological soul, we have new insight into mental disease, creativity, and the great artists of the present and from antiquity.

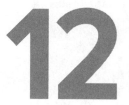

What Does the Future Hold?
Aging and the Future of the Biological Soul

All cities deteriorate with age. Buildings start to leak and crumble. Streets and sidewalks crack. Transportation and communication systems become slower and less reliable. This is as true for the "city" of your body as it is for the cities of the world. Sorry, there is no fountain of youth at the end of this book. If you are 65, so is your immune system. Your biological soul may want you to live to 100, but it will experience at least some senescence as you age, no matter how strong your immunity is now. That said, I love the way people refer to age as "just a number." This, in essence, is a true statement: All cities react differently to age and the rate of deterioration is worse in some than in others overall. Our immune systems are unique and much of how we age depends on how we live, our behavior, and our genetics. To put it another way, age *can* be relative; This is why even I sometimes cannot tell a 60-year-old from an 80-year-old in appearance and attitude.

The relativity of age and the uniqueness of the immune system make a chapter about its future a bit of an exercise in relativity as well. But I'm up for the challenge. For an immunologist like me, the question, *What does the future hold?* has dual meaning. Personally, I want to understand what is happening to my immune system as I age. Professionally, I revel in how much there is yet to understand about the biological soul, the mind-body connection, and human health and wellbeing overall. In this final chapter, I approach the question about the future from my personal and professional sides: first with a look at immune system senescence and what, if anything, you can do about it; and then with my predictions of what we might see in unraveling the mysteries of the biological soul.

IMMUNOSENESCENCE: OUR AGING FIRST RESPONDERS

There is no doubt that your immunity weakens with age. At no time was that more obvious than during the COVID-19 pandemic. People over 65, particularly those in nursing homes or in densely populated areas, succumbed quickly to the virus and were much more likely to die when infected than any other category of people. That's because when we get old, we have increased susceptibility to infectious diseases and a decreased response to vaccination, as your immune system might be a bit crotchety and unable to respond robustly to the boost. This decline is called immune system senescence, or immunosenescence—the process of gradual deterioration of our immune system because of age.

Immunosenescence has a major effect on your innate and adaptive immune response. When your thymus disappears after puberty, the output of naïve T lymphocytes and antigen experienced T cells accumulate. The T cell repertoire is fixed as highly differentiated effector T cells, and they produce more proinflammatory cytokines, which together with activated innate cells, contribute to a systemic inflammatory climate in older age. In other words, the cells—just like you—are getting older, and they might not be as up to their game as they were when you were 25, which is why there tends to be more inflammation with age. This edgy profile is just like the situation in the blood of women after giving birth; it is the body's way of maintaining some stability.

Immunosenescence usually coincides with the waning of your levels of sex steroid hormones, the decrease in healthy organisms in your biome, and the worsening of comorbidities like diabetes, dementia, and congestive heart failure, in addition to an overall decrease in the ability of your kidneys to clear toxins from the blood. Notice that I said "usually." Since every person is different, every person experiences this senescence differently and to different degrees. You might respond well to vaccines (as many did to the COVID-19 versions), be relatively free of comorbidities, and/or maintain your sex drive, libido, and biomes as you approach 100. Some of the variation depends on immunogenetics—the genetics of your immune system or what I called "regular inheritance" in Chapter 8. These genetics play a major role in how your immune system stays healthy as you age, particularly when it comes to your biological sex and the hormones you produce.

Hormones affect both men and women at the cellular and molecular level, and in general, the change of these individual hormones decrease optimal immune responses in both sexes.[1] But there are sexual *dimorphisms*—differences between male and female—regarding the response to infection, and not just when we become senior citizens. For example, sexually transmitted diseases occur more frequently and severely in women during their reproductive years due to behavior and sex-related mechanisms of reproduction but probably sex-specific steroid hormone levels as well. At menopause, the amount of estrogen in women drops, enhancing the immunosenescent effects of age, and placing postmenopausal women at significant risk of infection. There are receptors for female hormones on most cells of the innate and adaptive immune system, including many we have covered—natural killer

---

[1] Interestingly, there is some work being done at University of Alabama, showing that increased levels of hormones like leptin and insulin might protect humans in their 90s from immunosenescence.

T cells, B cells, white cells called macrophages, dendritic cells—and some we have not, like polymorphonuclear leukocytes. This is at least part of the reason aging women lose their immunological advantage and face increased susceptibility and mortality regarding many infections like hepatitis, meningitis, and pneumonia. Women also have more CD4 positive T cells and higher levels of the circulating antibodies, in particular, IgM, which probably adds to a woman's risk of autoimmune disease with age.

The effects of aging on men, however, can be just as startling, reflecting the lower levels of testosterone. Men experience a loss of energy, a mellowing of personality, and more risks for heart disease, hypertension, and stroke. Age-related changes in the immune system also occur more rapidly in men. Male hormone receptors have been identified on both T and B lymphocytes, and studies show age-related changes in lymphocyte subsets in elderly men, with the decline of T cells (including naïve CD4, CD8, CD28, B cells), T cell proliferative capacity, and cytokine IL-6 secretion. There are also weaker increases in memory and natural killer T cells. Certain cytokines are also decreased in men as they age, but not women. I suspect that the shorter life spans of men are related to these immune changes.

While age-related changes in sex steroid levels enhance immunosenescence-related alterations, women can reverse these aging changes by taking hormone replacement, a therapy not available to men. But as we learned, your biological sex is not the only kind of genetics that impact the immune system and immunosenescence. Epigenetics or "temporary inheritance" also plays a role here.

Many of the comorbidities we face are brought about by our behavior and the choices we make like smoking and alcohol, as I stated in Chapter 8. Smoking in Europe accounts for 60 percent of gender-specific mortality as well as many more cases of enhanced morbidity. Smoking is followed by alcohol abuse, risk-taking measures, and noncompliance with doctor's orders in the failure to support a normal immune system. If you thought tobacco smoking resulted in fewer deaths in the United States where there are more restrictions, you would be correct, but the effects from smoking still cause almost 500,000 deaths a year and remain the leading cause of cardiovascular disease (the leading cause of death in the country). Americans also drink too much, use illicit drugs, and take antibiotics and other medications in excess, and recent studies show binge drinking is up significantly with women. These risk factors and lifestyle choices interfere with the aging process and produce epigenetic effects that you do not want to pass down to the next generation.

Those next generations will surely be facing endemic and new criminal attacks on the cities of their bodies. In addition, the environment will change as the world warms and becomes more crowded, bringing new challenges. It is important that lawlessness be prevented, but even as we learn more about immunity and how antigens attack and create new treatments and vaccines, criminals will always find new ways to attack and avoid detection by the first responders sworn to protect us. But unlike the first responders of an actual city, we can't replace our body's first responders with new recruits. So, what can we do to help them as we age?

Beyond avoiding excessive negative behavior, there are positive ways to mitigate the aging process and manage your immune system, and we have covered many of them in this book: getting adequate sleep, maintaining a healthy biome, exercising, and sustaining sexual health if just from a nice hug every day, or even from a pet.

Exercise is of particular importance as we age. Remember: It does not mean running marathons or Spartan races. It needs to be a daily effort to work the body in favor of the biological soul—to let go, relax the brain, stress the body in a good way, and luxuriate in the flow of hormones, endorphins, and cytokines. Of equal importance are the mind-body connections to enhance immune function and immunity strength as we age, which bear repeating and cannot be understated, starting with relationships.

The American philosopher Henry David Thoreau famously moved to Walden Pond to live alone, meditate, and record natural observations he edited into his landmark 1854 book *Walden*. But he didn't pick the pond because he wanted to live as a hermit. Other people lived near the pond, Concord was less than a couple of miles away, and Boston less than 20. Even choosing to live alone, Thoreau knew the value of relationships if just to borrow an axe. We all had that need reaffirmed in the isolation of the COVID-19 pandemic. Zoom only does so much.

We need socialization and togetherness to make us happy *and* healthy. Loneliness has been linked to increased risk for heart disease and leads to huge increases in hospitalizations and ER visits. On the flip side, consider the Harvard Study of Adult Development, which since 1938 has tracked the lives of more than 700 men and found that the healthiest and happiest had the strongest relationships with others. Or consider the study of so-called blue zones of happiness, like Sardinia, Italy, and Loma Linda, California, where an unusually large number of people live to 100, have overall healthier lives, and suffer fewer diseases than other parts of the world. One of the biggest contributing factors to this longevity and one common to all the blue zones studied? Social interactions.

You can find these social interactions in the practices of meditation the way Thoreau never could. Standard meditative practice, Tai Chi, Qigong, or any other practice you find interesting are often done in groups, and this meditating will prolong your life by controlling the stresses that all of us face every day. Similarly, yoga has been shown to provide extensive relief of stress and pain; it's a great way to combine meditation with stretching and exercise to produce immune benefits if done with regularity. And since we have learned grief has an adverse effect on immunity, don't ignore the benefits of the power of positive thinking. I don't mean that if you believe you are better, you are. But there is some truth that you are only as sick as you act and think you are.

This power of positive thinking, however, may be all that is happening when it comes to trying to prevent immunosenescence through taking dietary additives like vitamins, holistic medications, and herbs to increase immune response.

DIETARY ADDITIVES

Many "immune strengthening" dietary additives and vitamins have ancient origins, but ironically, little hard data exists about their efficacy. Yet even without rigorous data to support their actions, many healthy people believe they would die without them and often bust their budgets to afford them. I am a scientist, so I have only limited recommendations for these additives, but I would be remiss if I didn't consider some of them—and any drawbacks—when it comes to immunity strong.

Let's start with vitamins. To be clear, *foods* that contain high levels of vitamins like A, C, D, and E, all support your immune system in different ways. For example, vitamin A—found in broccoli, carrots, sweet potatoes, and fortified milk—helps regulate the immune system and keeps tissue such as those of your lungs healthy. Other vitamins, such as C and E, have antioxidant potential, meaning they protect cells from oxidative stress or burning out from chemical exposures that oxidize and render your enzymes ineffective. You can find these vitamins in certain fish like salmon, sardines, and tuna, as well as Brazil nuts, walnuts, pumpkin seeds, mushrooms, whole grains, and many other plants.

Foods like sweet potatoes, dark chocolate, and berries of all sorts also provide antioxidants that the body uses to keep the immune system healthy and fend off diseases and infections. Garlic is a powerful antioxidant with antimicrobial, antiviral, and some say antibiotic properties. It's also a potent natural decongestant. Elderberry is packed with quercetin, an antioxidant with antihistamine and anti-inflammatory effects; a teaspoonful of elderberry syrup is used to combat flu symptoms and help people with sinus pain or chronic fatigue find relief. Spices such as turmeric, ginger, and garlic have major antioxidant and anti-inflammatory properties, too. Some data may be soft around these effects, but they are all delicious and nutritious, so add them away to your diet!

I cannot offer the same enthusiasm for adding vitamins in pill form. Outside of consumption of vitamins naturally, the only one

I recommend a supplement for is vitamin D. Many humans are deficient in vitamin D. We get it from (sensible exposure to) sunlight and foods like salmon, sardines, trout, and other fatty fish and fortified foods like milk and some cereals. As I touched on in Chapter 2, vitamin D has a powerful role in stimulating the immune system. It is particularly helpful in the destruction of viruses and other disease-causing invaders, which is why many physicians measure and replace it routinely. Vitamin D replacement only gains importance as we get older. It is associated with bone health, and we give it to patients along with calcium to control osteoporosis (bleaching of bone) due to aging, the ingestion of medications, or lack of sunlight, which was all too common during the early days of the pandemic and winter months in northern climes.

While many of my patients take vitamins in spite of my feelings, almost every other patient that I see in my clinic takes herbs or holistic medicines of some kind. Some of them tell me that they are better at keeping them healthier than their prescriptive medicines. Many of these herbs have been taken for centuries and their use is widely accepted by health-conscious people, and there is data that immunosuppressive herbs may work well for people who are taking medications for cancer because antioxidants make cancer cells multiply faster. In addition, some healthy plants like milk thistle, ginseng, green tea, black cumin, and licorice have been shown to be stimulants to immune health. But consult with your doctor before using any of them, because a few of them can have untoward effects, like licorice raising your blood pressure.

To consider every herb and natural medicine I have encountered would require another book, not to mention a degree in herbology. So, I am focusing on some that keep coming up, favored for their supposed ability to increase immune response.

You will see that China is the origin for these herbs and natural medicine, and many of the other holistic medications that are involved as alternative agents that strengthen the immune system. If you recall, I first visited China in 1989 and revisited several times after and saw how dedicated Chinese culture is to healing plans that can involve a combination of herbal therapy, acupuncture, and dietary changes with lifestyle shifts as much as modern medicine. I have no reason to dispute Chinese medicine or centuries of Chinese culture, but some of it is anecdotal and circumstantial. I'll never forget one early trip to China, where traditional doctors took me to snake dinner in Guangzhou (that's snake as in python, not steak as in cow—and they killed the snake at the table to show it was fresh!). The snake was supposed to protect against arthritis, because . . . no one had ever seen an arthritic snake. So, again, there is not a lot of scientific data around the following herbs and natural medicine that I have been asked about and some explicit warnings.

- *Echinacea*: An antiviral and antibacterial herb that contains polysaccharides, which increase the body's production of neutrophils, those cells that fight off infections (mostly bacterial) by consuming germs and carting them away like paddy wagons. Some of my patients take echinacea when they feel a cold coming on and others simply ingest the tablets daily to prevent viral infections like influenza or COVID-19. But know that there is *no* evidence that such an herb works on coronaviruses.
- *Bupleurum*: An herb that has been used in traditional Chinese medicine for centuries to "bring the body back to harmony." (Chinese practitioners believe that harmony resides in the liver, stomach, and spleen.) It is an immunosuppressant herb used to help with the treatment of certain cancers, gastrointestinal disorders, and liver disease. It can suppress the immune system and is also a diuretic and laxative. But many diuretics and laxative herb compounds are not only immunosuppressive, but can also deplete stores of minerals called electrolytes like potassium and make the body more susceptible to irregularities of the heart. Again, please consult your doctor.
- *Astragalus*: An herb thought to combat stress. The Chinese use this to fight fatigue and boost the immune system, especially during cold and flu season. It is highly possible that this was

an alternative medication that was used during COVID-19 in Wuhan, China.

- *Yin Chiao* (*honeysuckle forsythia*): A nine-herb formula used in China that contains a soothing licorice, nasal-clearing peppermint, perspiration-stimulating Jing Jie and Lu Jen that apparently soothe the lungs and the stomach.
- *Andrographis*: A plant commonly used in Asian countries to prevent influenza and soothe digestive issues, liver conditions, fever, and sore throats. Specifically directed to enhance the immune system, it is often used in China to fight infections.
- *Red yeast rice*: A fermented yeast product traditionally used as food coloring in Asian cuisine. It has been used by the Chinese for centuries and apparently is a drug that works as an immunosuppressant. The downside of using red yeast rice is that it could cause toxicity to the liver and should never be taken with alcohol or in combination with statin drugs (agents that lower cholesterol).
- *Cascara sagrada* or *yellow bark*: A natural stimulant laxative used to relieve constipation. The herb is generally considered safe for short-term use, but it can increase one's likelihood to get infections, become dehydrated, and develop low electrolytes and heart problems. It can also cause muscle weakness if used for more than a couple of days. The Brigham and Women's Hospital of Harvard University suggests that the immune system can become compromised when this stimulant is used for extended periods and could lead to cancer.
- *Glucosamine* or *glucosamine sulfate*: A chemical present in the fluid surrounding joints throughout the body. The natural form of glucosamine comes from shellfish, but it can be created in the laboratory. It is used widely to treat osteoarthritis and it supposedly has immunosuppressive qualities.

I could go on. Ginger, a pungent root, is a powerful antihistamine and decongestant that delivers a one-two punch against cold symptoms. Or maybe mushrooms—practitioners have used them for centuries, blending shiitake, reishi, and meatpacking mushrooms that are specifically directed to strengthen the immune system. And no discussion about holistic medicines would be complete without talking about anti-inflammatory agents. *Arnica* is used after trauma to decrease inflammation, and people are known to ingest it for musculoskeletal pains like a sore back. *Bromelain* from pineapple decreases inflammation by controlling pain and swelling. And, finally, there are compounds from ancient Indian Ayurveda medicine that stabilize and decrease stress and inflammation called *ashwagandha*, which is said to boost host resistance, decrease stress, and stabilize the body's balance.

What to make of all this? It is hard to say. Dr. Lahita says natural remedies without known side effects are the best to take, and there are many that have none and are inexpensive. Your physician should know that which you are taking for your good health. Dr. Bob believes these efforts to strengthen the immune system have been around for millennia in many cases before anyone knew that there was such a thing as the immune system. What is clear is the people offering them and taking them had an idea that there was a soul, perhaps biological, that needed care and nurturing and was of major importance to health and wellbeing. Perhaps the future will show us how right they were and how much more we still have to learn.

WHAT THE FUTURE HOLDS: PREDICTIONS FOR THE STUDY OF THE BIOLOGICAL SOUL

Many of us are and will continue to live beyond 100 years, which is not even a bold prediction. Life expectancy continues to increase around the world, and the United States has the largest number of centenarians (nearly 100,000 as I wrote this book) followed by Japan (though Japan has the largest number per capita). Yet for all we have talked about when it comes to what happens in the immune system, why it happens, and what can help and hurt it, there is still so much we can understand and learn. I predict that the immune system will give us much information over the next 25 years and many more people around the world will live healthier and far beyond age 100. Here are my boldest predictions, starting with ones related to behavior.

Depression, schizophrenia, and other mental disorders can be controlled by our understanding of the immune system: COVID-19 taught us that viral infection of the brain and the long-haul syndrome involving suicides from depression, the beginnings of paranoid schizophrenia, and overall changes in personality exist long after a viral infection. Add this to the established fact that the immune system is abnormal in many patients with mental illnesses, and scientists will establish an immunological basis for diseases and disorders once thought purely neurological. It is possible that we will be using anti-cytokine treatments instead of antipsychotics in the near future to treat mental diseases.

Behavioral conditions and neurodevelopmental abnormalities can be predicted and controlled through our understanding of immune regulation: The growth of the brain's hemispheres will be shown to relate to what you do in later life. We will see connections and learn about new relationships between autism and neurodevelopmental conditions like ADHD, word blindness, and dyslexia and immunological dysregulation, the influence of the maternal immune system, and environmental stress.

New understandings will emerge as to how the immune system plays a role in handedness and creativity: That the brain and the immune system develop together and whether hormones like fetal levels of testosterone that neurologists say cause enlargement of the right side of the brain will remain of great interest to embryologists and neuroscientists. The legitimate but controversial issues regarding handedness, creativity, and sexual preference could lead to a development of ways to engineer talents through our knowledge of the brain's immune system.

Long-haul syndromes reveal secrets about our bodies: Until COVID-19, we had never considered on any scale the idea that the immune system could be tricked to produce disease symptoms—heart disease, inflamed lungs, new clotting mechanisms, muscle weakness, chronic shortness of breath—and that these symptoms could be evidence of post-viral disease. We had, of course, known every one of these symptoms and more before, but never attributed them to a virus. COVID-19 brought this possibility crashing down on medicine with such rapidity that we barely had time to digest the pathology that was found in patients many months—and now more than a year—after the initial infection. Time will give us the chance to examine enough patients to understand what happened and treat these effects and further probe the depths of our biological soul.

Discovery that inflammation and infection within the brain might be a root cause and a path to fighting dementia: Chronic immune conditions and COVID-19 long-haul effects include "foggy brain," loss of memory, delusions, and hallucinations. Our understanding of brain inflammation and the brain's immune response to infection will result in an understanding of dementia and a possible vaccine or immune or cytokine intervention to prevent it. A lot of signs and laboratory parameters in people with dementia point to inflammation and possible infection as precursors for the disease. (Amyloid protein is one associated with dementia like Alzheimer's disease.)

Checkpoint immunological treatment of cancer will include the most resistant tumors: The many cancers that are beginning to be approached immunologically when the protection proteins and antibodies that keep the cancer safe are removed will lead to a way to attack tumors in even the most privileged sites and those cancers that were usually resistant to treatment. Proteins are present that prevent the immune system from rejecting an obvious malignancy in the body. Chimeric antigen receptor

T cell therapy (Car T cells) is a way to get these immune cells designed to attack certain cancers through training in the lab for leukemia, lymphoma, and possibly multiple myeloma. These will be new uses of adaptive immunity to fight diseases. Most exciting is the use of immune checkpoints to treat heretofore resistant cancers along with standard radiation and chemotherapy to take on difficult cancers like pancreas, which usually fail to respond to treatment.

Asthma, eczema, and other neonatal conditions will be prevented by influencing the fetal immune system throughout pregnancy: I like to think of this as the evolution of creative learning in the womb. Science shows that you can influence your baby's behavior and future by paying close attention to yourself while pregnant: Stay healthy, take no medicines if possible, and eat well. The baby is a transplant and depends on your body for nourishment to create the biome for the baby's future. A mother's immune system will nurture the baby for several months and the neonate's immune system will begin to mature while the neonate is still in the womb. Once delivered, the flora or the vagina will give a new spark to the biome developing within the baby and influence the kinds of diseases and possible behavioral traits the baby will have while she or he grows. The baby's breastfeeding is also a plus for the developing biome.

Your innate and adaptive immune system can be taught to control autoimmunity: Today's molecular miracles are already influencing the future of immunity. As a result, we should be able to control autoimmunity that causes disease by learning about the triggers that cause such autoimmune diseases as rheumatoid arthritis, lupus, and many more. Anti-cytokine and anti-chemokine biological drugs are now in development for almost every immune disease, and the data will show that these biologicals will be useful to control B and T cells' influence on autoimmunity. We are also finally beginning to appreciate that the signals and triggers for many of the diseases that are caused by epigenetic influences, such as diet, environment, exposure to viruses, and rogue bacteria, that can be passed down to future generations. Finally, we will develop a way to understand each person's immunogenetics, so we know who is and who is not susceptible to (the bad effects of) viruses.

Epigenetic influences on race and immunity and overall health will be addressed: In 2021, following the ravages of the COVID-19 pandemic that disproportionately affected non-Caucasian populations, the head of the Centers for Disease Control and Prevention ranked racism as a major threat to public health. Different health outcomes for different races have been documented for years. Having more doctors who look like the populations they treat will help mitigate this, but so will understanding that these effects are epigenetic or temporary inheritance rather than genetic or regular inheritance and are reversible.

Vaccines will be ready for future pandemics: The foray into messenger RNA COVID-19 vaccines is a quantum leap forward with regard to safe and quick biological protection. In the future, computerized machines will analyze the genomes (DNA or RNA) of organisms within minutes and then identify the sweet spots of an infective antigen. As a result, we should be able to make new vaccines in weeks rather than months or years. This will also be true for the quick inoculation against variants of endemic diseases, which COVID-19 also taught us.

Oral medicines will inhibit replication of viruses like COVID-19: Ongoing efforts to develop oral drugs to inhibit replication of viruses like COVID-19 will be successful, inhibiting the RNA replicase enzyme within infected cells and prohibit the virus's multiplication and development. These pills will supersede the vaccines and will be analogous to Tamiflu for influenza or Sofosbuvir for hepatitis C.

Inflammation and infection will be recognized as being at the core of common causes of death: We know that inflammation and clotting are two processes that influence longevity. We also know that atherosclerosis is enhanced in some immune diseases like rheumatoid arthritis and lupus. Can we use this information to control atherosclerosis and its attendant illnesses? Can we understand that inflammation is at the core of our most common diseases, and indirectly, the immune system? Is the stimulation of the immune system through infection conducive to the inflammatory processes that cause atherosclerosis, heart disease, and stroke? We have learned much from the pandemic in this regard, and I believe that immunity is at the core of these diseases.

We will define the biome of aging people: There is a belief that the biome of all organs, but especially that of the bowel, changes with age, and not for the better. In the future, we should be able to change the flora of the bowel and the skin to use bacteria for long life and preservation of immunity. It might even be possible to roll aging back with an altered population of organisms resemblant of a 20-year-old.

Intimacy and immune function will be forever linked: We know about oxytocin, the love hormone that is produced in large amounts by the very act of embracing and loving someone, and we know that prolactin, the "milk-releasing hormone," is important as an immune enhancer. The act of intercourse will be forever known as a big boost to the immune system because of the showers of pleasurable hormones, cytokines, and endorphins that result.

DR. BOB SAYS

Ending on that prediction was intentional. It allows me to say one more time that so much of who we are and will become when it comes to our health and happiness depends on our relationships and how we treat others, not just ourselves.

LET YOUR SOUL SHINE

Every living creature has a protective system that is their immunity. In us, our immune system is so physically and spiritually profound that I call it our biological soul. Every one of us—regardless of sex, race, ethnicity, religion, or political belief—has one. It is the compass that takes us to the end of life—taking all we give it, the good and the bad, to keep us ticking, so to speak. Science has given us understandings of the immune system, cell biology, and the influence of bacteria and viruses that allow us insights into every organ and disease mechanism, paths to create new vaccines in ways never done before, and ways to beat cancers and even disorders of the brain. These understandings and our marvelous responses to them are tailored by thousands of years of inheritance from countless relatives over generations—the basis for your biological soul, each as different as the shapes of sand grains on a beach. This is what makes us unique and unites us at the same time. This is Immunity Strong, the true essence of being human.

Glossary

This glossary is not designed to be comprehensive, nor could it ever be. It reviews some of the key terms used in the text, as well as some additional terms we did not cover in depth, but you might encounter on Dr. Google and beyond as you further explore the idea of "immunity strong."

Acute phase reactants: Proteins that circulate in the blood and are elevated in inflammation.

Adaptive immune response: The response of lymphocytes that are specific to a particular antigen. This involves immunologic memory, or recognition of the foreign antigen. The key to this kind of immunity is the establishment of clones of lymphocytes against a specific target antigen.

Adjuvant: A substance that strengthens the immune response. Usually administered with a vaccine. An example of an adjuvant is aluminum hydroxide.

Alarmin: Part of an effective response to viruses, bacteria within cells, and parasites—albeit primitive, as it is said to be a remnant of primitive immunity and present in many other species besides humans. It recognizes microbes based on patterns of recognition.

Allergic reaction: The body's response to an antigen or foreign substance, resulting in increased abnormal activity of the immune system. This might be an immediate reaction to plant pollen, insect toxin, components of food, or a medicine.

Allergy: A condition induced by a foreign substance. The antibody that responds to this foreigner is a specific kind of antibody called IgE. Cells that are involved in an allergy are eosinophils and mast cells.

Antibodies: Proteins in the blood made by plasma cells, which are descended from B cells. These are the arresting officers of the immune system. Another name for antibodies is immunoglobulins and there are several types: IgG, M, E, D, and A. These are made specifically to lock around the foreign substance like handcuffs, allowing the criminal to be eaten by the phagocytes and carried off to the spleen.

Anticancer antibodies: Cells directed against tumors or malignant tissue.

Antigen: The criminal, usually a foreign substance (virus, bacteria, or parasite), that the immune system addresses in many ways. In autoimmunity, the antigen can be a person's own tissues (blood cells, platelets, skin, etc.). In allergic responses, it can be a peanut, pollen, or medicine that becomes the foreigner after the immune system reviews its presence.

Antigen-Presenting Cells (APC): Cells also known as macrophages, dendritic cells, and B cells that are able to engulf a foreign substance in the process of arresting them for invading the body. Once engulfed, the antigen is digested into fragments, which are then presented to the receptors on T cells (the detective division of the body's police). Based on the genetic identifier (MHC) of the arrest, these cells present the criminal to the appropriate cells for recognition for later encounters.

Antigen receptors: The whole process of arrest and criminal recognition begins with these receptors. Found on B and T cells and coded by different genes, these receptors are critical for the immune system's recognition of an antigen or a fragment of an antigen.

Anti-inflammatory drugs: Medicines that inhibit inflammatory processes.

Autoantibodies: Antibodies or proteins which are directed at "self," meaning your own cells and tissues.

Autoantigens: Cells and tissues that are part of your body that are mistaken as foreign by the immune system.

Autoimmune diseases: Diseases caused by the body's immune system reacting with "self" antigens such as a heart valve, platelets, or the kidneys. Diseases might be rheumatic fever, lupus, rheumatoid arthritis, or multiple sclerosis.

Autoimmunity: The process giving rise to unregulated immune reactions against a person's own bodily tissues.

Bacteria: Single-cell organisms that can be either aerobic (living with oxygen) or anaerobic (living without oxygen). They make up the biomes of the body along with fungi and parasites.

B cells: Cells that mature in the bone marrow and receive their orders from a variety of other cells. After stimulation by a foreign substance, these cells become plasma cells, which produce antibodies. These are the rank-and-file police of the immune system and they use antibodies to "snare" the bad guys.

Biological: A medicine that is not a drug, but a substance like a monoclonal antibody.

Biome: Collections of organisms in the bowel, on the skin, or in organs like the lung that have their own ecology and are generally supportive of us as hosts. They are essential to informing the immune system of self or nonself and increase the overall efficiency of things like vaccines.

Blood-brain barrier: The border between the brain and spinal cord and the rest of the body. It is a filtration site, patrolled by certain T cells and other cells of the monocyte families. It prevents infection of the brain or movement of toxins into the brain space.

Complement: A series of sugar-proteins found on the surface of cells and free in the blood. They often do damage to invading organisms and "complement" the immune reaction.

Carcinogen: Any cancer-causing agent in the environment.

CD (cluster of differentiation): A set of surface markers that designate types of cells, their source, and how they should interact with other cells. It is the marker on the roof of the police vehicle, paddy wagon, or detective unit.

Cellular immunity: Immunity involving the cells of the immune system.

Chemokine: A large group of proteins that tell cells where to go like a 911 call.

Chromosomes: Threadlike structure in the nucleus of cells that carries genetic material and information in the form of genes made up of DNA and wrapped in proteins.

C-reactive protein: An acute phase reactant and a good marker of inflammation anywhere in the body.

CRISPR: A technique of editing genes using bacterial enzymes to slice and splice parts of the human genome.

Cytokine: Communication molecules produced by cells of the immune system that tells cells what to do. They function as local hormones, influence the duration of an immune and inflammatory response, and are thought to have effects beyond that of the immune system. Each cytokine is given a number and can be followed within the body. They exist everywhere, even the brain. Also called interleukin.

Cytotoxic cells: Cells that damage or kill. They can be specific depending on immune instruction and they can eliminate a foreign invader. When they are cytotoxic (cell toxic) T cells, they can surround and kill cells infected with a virus.

Defensins: Substances within the innate immune system that are specifically directed to viruses or bacteria and capable of killing them. Called pattern recognition receptors, they are found in macrophages and white cells and can react and destroy any cells in the body.

Dendritic cells: Sophisticated cells that present the antigens to the immune system and are usually part of the innate immune response. They respond without concern about the nature of the invader. Their job is to find, identify, recognize the foreigner, and alert everyone else. They are present in various organs and have their own identity.

DNA: A sugar backbone in the form of a double helix, consisting of specific chemical bases in combination called nucleotides. All of our regular inherited genetic information is in our DNA. There are four bases that in various combinations constitute your genes. The bases are adenine, cytosine, guanine, or thymine.

DNA virus: A virus in which the genetic material within it is DNA. Examples are herpes, smallpox, and adenovirus.

Eosinophils: White blood cells activated by the cells of the adaptive immune response chiefly against parasites.

Erythrocytes: Red blood cells.

Freund's adjuvant: A substance which enhances an antigen and made of dried TB bacteria. Only used to augment the immune response in animals. It is not used in humans.

Gene: The basic units of heredity on chromosomes.

Gene expression: The information passed on from the gene. The gene is transcribed in the nucleus of the cell and then translated by messenger RNA outside of the nucleus in a part of the cell called the cytoplasm. The mRNA then makes proteins.

Genes for T cell receptors: Genes that make the T cell receptor—a very specific receptor that determines the immune response of T cells.

Genome: The sets of genes within a cell, bacteria, or virus that have the formula for the expression of certain proteins. This is the term for the entire map of heredity in each animal, plant, or individual, specific to that individual.

Granulocytes: Another name for white blood cells. They make up 70 percent of the cells in the blood.

Helper T cells: One set of T cells that induce the immune response. These are the detectives of the immune system. They have a marker on their surface called CD4, which I liken to the numbers on the roofs of police cars that can only be seen from above.

Histocompatibility: The compatibility of tissues from another individual (basically the ability of tissues to get along with one another). The compatibility is determined by the antigens on both the donor and the recipient's tissues.

HLA (human leukocyte antigens): Antigens important to the establishment of histocompatibility between two people.

Histone: Proteins around which DNA wraps in the nucleus of the cell.

Homeostasis: Biological equilibrium within the body, when everything is working well.

Hormones: Regulatory chemical messengers that signal cells and tissues to do certain functions. They can be made in specific organs like the pancreas, the ovary, testicle, and thyroid, and travel in the blood to signal an organ or group of cells to turn on or off.

Hybridoma: A cell population derived from a fusion of two different cells from the same person. Fusion of a B cell with a myeloma cancer cell allows the development of a single clone of cells capable of making copious amounts of a specific antibody called monoclonal.

Immunoglobulins: Antibodies or proteins in the blood with structures that allow them to react with antigens and form antigen-antibody combinations called immune complexes.

Interleukin: Another name for more than over 200 cytokines produced by white cells.

Immune complexes: A circulating complex of antibodies and antigens. They usually wreak havoc as sources of inflammation and are the source of much pain, discomfort, and tissue destruction in the body.

Immune response: A response to a foreign agent. First the innate or immediate response and then the adaptive immunity or immunity based on antigen recognition.

Immunity: The protective system within your body.

Immunization: Getting a specific weak antigen in any number of ways to provoke your immune system to protect you. Today, injection of nucleic acid like mRNA or DNA can shortcut the need for weak antigens and make selected antigens in cells that mimic that of an actual infection.

Immunodeficiencies: Absence either by hereditary or (purposely) via medication of a critical arm of the immune system. They can be antibody deficiency or deficiencies of cells like T cells.

Immunogenetics: The study of the inheritance of the immune system (antigens of the MHC, antibodies, receptors, and various cells).

Immunologic memory: The ability of your B and T cell first responders to respond to foreign substances that they remember.

Immunologic tolerance: When the immune system no longer responds to a specific antigen, and the response is suppressed.

Immunomodulation: Controlling the immune system, either through stimulation or suppression.

Inflammation: Reaction of the body to cellular injury. The goal is to eliminate the harmful factor and repair the damaged area. It is the biological equivalent of a crime scene.

Innate or nonspecific immune response: Immunity that occurs right after the body is in contact with a foreign agent, usually an infectious agent like a bacterium or a virus. It is essentially the SWAT team of the immune system.

Interferons: Cytokines produced by different cells that are critical to resist viral infection. The main interferon molecules are antiviral.

Interleukins: Another name for cytokines or communication molecules.

Killer cells: T cells that can kill other cells infected with specific markers on their surface. Also known as a cytotoxic T cell.

Leukocytes: White blood cells.

Long haul: A term given to patients who have suffered infection after the elimination of the organism. It refers specifically to disability that is often prolonged and said to be the result of an immune response without the antigen.

Lymph nodes: Nodes that are strategically situated throughout the body like openings around the anus, genitals, oral cavity, particularly places where organisms might be likely to enter. I like to compare these to police precincts within the body.

Lymphocyte: The principal cells of the immune system.

Macrophage: Antigen-presenting cells present in various organs of the body and the major aspect of the innate immune response and crucial to your defenses. They are also important in antibody immunity and cellular immunity.

Major histocompatibility complex (MHC): A cluster of genes on chromosome 6 whose products are transplantation antigens. The molecules of the MHC can regulate the immune response. It makes proteins involved in antigen processing and other aspects of host defense. Many variations of this gene cluster occur throughout the genome and are specific to you.

Mast cell: White cells that have a crucial role in allergic reactions. Like eosinophils, they can release granules that cause allergic reactions.

Memory cells: B or T lymphocytes that are produced after the first contact with a specific antigen and remember it. They can then recall the antigen and respond rapidly when rechallenged by it.

Messenger RNA (mRNA): Single-stranded RNA molecules that specify the amino acid sequence for one or more proteins. It carries information from genes to ribosomes where it is made into proteins.

Messenger RNA (mRNA) vaccine: Use of a selected mRNA fraction of a virus injected into people as a vaccine to produce specific proteins on the surface of a cell and make the body think that it has been infected.

Monoclonal antibodies: Identical copies of antibody molecules that have specific combining sites directed against a single part of foreign antigen. They are the result of the growth of tumor plasma cells and can be made under artificial laboratory conditions using technology called hybridoma. Most of the new biological drugs we use to treat everything from arthritis to cancer to COVID-19 are monoclonal antibodies.

Monocyte: A large cell making up to 10 percent of the total white cell count in people. When it gets into tissues, it develops into a tissue macrophage.

Neutrophil: A white cell that constitutes 45 to 70 percent of the total white cells in the blood. They are the paddy wagons of the immune system as they often scoop up and eat foreign substances and they can also engulf material designated as foreign by other cells of the immune system.

Natural killer cells: Five to ten percent of the total lymphocyte counts in the peripheral blood. In addition to B and T lymphocytes, these cells represent the third major subpopulation of cells. They mainly kill tumor cells and virus-infected cells. Also called cytotoxic T cells.

Parasite: Any number of worms, liver flukes, and one-cell animals that use the body as a source of nutrition.

Phagocytes: Neutrophils or macrophages able to engulf or inactivate particles or organisms. These cells scoop foreign material up and take it to the spleen or to lymph nodes.

Plasma cells: Cells that produce and secrete antibodies. They become plasma cells from B lymphocytes that are stimulated by antigens.

Platelets: Particles that are essential to blood clotting.

Polyclonal antibodies: Large groups of conventional antibodies that are found in the blood.

Proinflammatory: Agents that stimulate inflammation.

Receptor: The way cells communicate. Usually located on the cell surface, they can be blocked and are used by hormones, cytokines, and other molecules for intra-immune communication.

Sepsis: Infection of the body by bacteria. It can also be a serious condition in which bacterial toxins get into the body blood and cause shock.

Shock: A generalized reaction of the body to sudden and strong stimuli from either the external or internal environment. It is manifested by, among others, a reduction of blood pressure and the beginning of respiratory problems. Shock can be the result of trauma, hemorrhage, or failure of the heart and the lungs. But it is usually the effect of toxins from infective agents like bacteria.

Spleen: The prison of the body, or the place where criminal antigens are deposited whole or in part by cells of the immune system, typically phagocytes.

T lymphocytes: Cells that have been developed in the thymus and acquire competence as the detective division of the immune system. The surface marker for these T cells is CD4. These comprise a heterogeneous population. There are helper T cells called TH1 or TH2. TH1 cells make cytokines and are proinflammatory cells that get macrophages excited. TH2 cells also make cytokines but they order B cells to begin making antibody.

T lymphocyte, cytotoxic: A subpopulation of T lymphocytes that carry a surface receptor called CD8. T cells called cytotoxic have a major role in killing cells infected by viruses or other parasites, to attack tumor-transformed cells/cells that are malignant.

T lymphocytes, helper: T cells with a surface receptor called CD4. They usually help B lymphocytes in recognizing criminals.

T lymphocytes, suppressor: T cells that suppress immune reactions.

Thymus gland: Primarily an organ in which T lymphocytes mature and differentiate in order to recognize foreign antigens. It's essentially a training school for detectives and has its own training staff called thymocytes.

Tumor necrosis factor (TNF): A very potent cytokine within the body that acts as a cytotoxin. There are many monoclonal antibodies (like Remicade, Enbrel, and Humira) that are available to inhibit this particular cytokine.

Vaccine: Using nucleic acids or attenuated or dead microorganisms to stimulate the formation of specific antibodies or T cell responses to protect us from the bad deeds of microorganisms.

Vasculitis: Inflammation of a blood vessel wall of any diameter that results in death of cells.

Virus: Infectious dead particles that can use cells to replicate.

Acknowledgments

This work would not be possible without the following individuals.

The first is Jim Eber, who is nothing short of a genius. The development and organization of the book is clearly an unrelenting series of creative suggestions and moves suggested by him. Numerous late-night meetings and Zoom calls clarified much and made the book more readable than I ever expected.

Claudia Riemer Boutote at Red Raven Studio, my agent, is the person who believed in this work and pushed me forward with helpful suggestions. She tirelessly gave me instructions, worked, and reworked my writing in the beginning to engineer a brilliant proposal for the book during the pandemic.

Mary Glenn, my publisher, and deputy publisher Keith Pfeffer deserve credit for having faith in my ability to write this book in a short period of time. Their patience and grace allowed me to work on this book with the hope that it would be a successful read.

I thank my many colleagues at the Rockefeller University Hospital during this terrible pandemic, as well as the colleagues who supported my ideas listed throughout the text. I also thank the many patients who stimulated discussions and are occasionally used as examples.

I cannot thank enough the late Henry G. Kunkel MD, my mentor and professor, who inspired my education in immunology. His guidance allowed me to write for textbooks and edit my own. He was truly the father of modern immunology and my own scientific father. I also owe my interest in writing to the late Professor Lewis Thomas, with whom I worked for many years. "Uncle Lou" wrote about everything and took notes every day for his many books. He was also a free thinker who embraced every idea.

Last but never least, to my lovely wife and partner, the great artist Carolyn D. Palmer: Thank you for always supporting this effort, providing me with creative and spiritual energy, and coming up with the idea that anchors the whole book: the biological soul.

Index

About the Author

Robert G. Lahita, MD, PhD ("Dr. Bob"), is a professor of medicine at Hackensack Meridian School of Medicine and clinical professor of medicine at Rutgers New Jersey Medical School. He is also the director of the Institute for Autoimmune and Rheumatic Disease at St. Joseph's Health in Paterson, New Jersey. Prior to his current work, Dr. Bob was chair of medicine at St. Joseph's Medical Center, Newark Beth Israel Medical Center, and Jersey City Medical Center and was division director of rheumatic disease for many years at St. Luke's Roosevelt Hospital in New York City. He also served as division chief of rheumatology at Saint Vincent Hospital in New York City and Professor at NYMC. He has trained countless medical students, residents, and fellows during his career.

Dr. Bob received his MD and PhD in Microbiology and Molecular Genetics from Jefferson Medical College and Thomas Jefferson University in Philadelphia. His research interests have always been in the field of autoimmunity and immunoendocrinology, and he proudly served as an associate professor in immunology for 11 years in the laboratory of the legendary Henry G.

Kunkel at The Rockefeller University in New York City. While at Rockefeller, he was an adjunct professor at Weill Cornell Medical School. For more than a decade, he was also an associate professor at Columbia University.

Dr. Bob has also had an interest in emergency medicine and has been the volunteer medical director for the Ridgewood, New Jersey, Emergency Services for more than 30 years and served as the police surgeon and fire department medical director. He is also the medical director of Saddle River, New Jersey, and vice chair of the Board of Health. During the 9/11 tragedy, Dr. Bob was part-time medical director of Hudson County, New Jersey, and played a significant role on the New Jersey side of the Hudson River and at "Ground Zero."

Dr. Bob is a Master of the American College of Rheumatology, a Fellow of the American College of Physicians, and the Royal College of Physicians (London). He has been editor or associate editor of several medical journals, the author of more than 150 scientific papers, and written or edited 14 books, including *Systemic Lupus Erythematosus*, which is now in its sixth edition. In 2004, he received a Doctor of Humane Letters from St. Peter's University, Honoris Causa.

Dr. Bob has been a frequent guest on television networks, including Newsmax, Fox Business, Fox News, NBC Now, MSNBC, EWTN and CBSN and was consulted constantly during the COVID-19 pandemic by those networks and media across the globe.

An accomplished accordionist, Dr. Bob is married to the renowned sculptor and artist, Carolyn D. Palmer. He has two sons and two grandchildren.

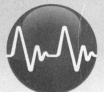

Simple **Heart Test**

Powered by Newsmaxhealth.com

FACT:

▸ Nearly half of those who die from heart attacks each year never showed prior symptoms of heart disease.

▸ If you suffer cardiac arrest outside of a hospital, you have just a 7% chance of survival.

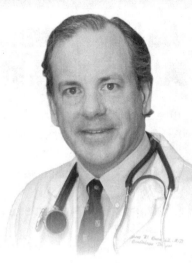

Don't be caught off guard. Know your risk now.

TAKE THE TEST NOW ...

Renowned cardiologist **Dr. Chauncey Crandall** has partnered with **Newsmaxhealth.com** to create a simple, easy-to-complete, online test that will help you understand your heart attack risk factors. Dr. Crandall is the author of the #1 best-seller *The Simple Heart Cure: The 90-Day Program to Stop and Reverse Heart Disease.*

Take Dr. Crandall's Simple Heart Test — it takes just 2 minutes or less to complete — it could save your life!

Discover your risk now.

- **Where you score on our unique heart disease risk scale**
- Which of your lifestyle habits really protect your heart
- **The true role your height and weight play in heart attack risk**
- Little-known conditions that impact heart health
- Plus much more!

SimpleHeartTest.com/711

Allergy-Proof Your Life

Natural Remedies for Allergies That Work!

Allergy-Proof Your Life

NATURAL REMEDIES FOR ALLERGIES THAT WORK!

✓ Asthma ✓ Nutritional deficiencies

✓ Seasonal allergies ✓ Itching & Hives

✓ Rashes & Eczema ✓ Congestion

✓ Inflammation ✓ Sinusitis

✓ Leaky or inflamed gut ✓ Rhinitis

Inside Delicious Recipes for Allergy Relief

Michelle Schoffro Cook, PhD, DNM, ROHP
Award-Winning and Bestselling Natural Health Author

Inside *Allergy-Proof Your Life*:

- ✓ **What You Should Never, Ever Eat if You Suffer From Allergies**
- ✓ Dangers and Limitations of Common Allergy Medications
- ✓ **Top Foods & Nutrients to Help You Fight Allergies**
- ✓ The Gut-Allergy Connection Your Doctor Won't Tell You About
- ✓ **And Much More . . .**

FREE OFFER

Claim Your FREE OFFER Now!

Claim your **FREE** copy of *Allergy-Proof Your Life* — a **$24.99 value** — today with this special offer. Just cover $4.95 for shipping & handling.

Plus, you will receive a bonus **FREE** report — *Over-the-Counter Health Hazards* — from one of America's foremost holistic physicians, David Brownstein, M.D.

We'll also send you a 3-month risk-free trial subscription to **Dr. David Brownstein's Natural Way to Health** which provides you with the most recent insights on emerging natural treatments along with the best of safe conventional medical care.

"*Allergy-Proof Your Life* is a great resource for all allergy sufferers. It helps you discover the underlying causes of your allergies, so you can heal them once and for all."
— *Dr. Brownstein, M.D.*

Get Your FREE Copy of *Allergy-Proof* TODAY!

Newsmax.com/Immunity